Relieving Headaches and Migraines

David Hazard

HARVEST HOUSE PUBLISHERS
Eugene, Oregon 97402

Cover by Left Coast Design, Portland, Oregon

Advisory

Readers are advised to consult with their physician or other medical practitioner before implementing the suggestions that follow.

This book is not intended to take the place of sound medical advice or to treat specific maladies. Neither the author nor the publisher assumes any liability for possible adverse consequences as a result of the information contained herein.

RELIEVING HEADACHES AND MIGRAINES
Copyright © 2002 by David Hazard
Published by Harvest House Publishers
Eugene, Oregon 97402

Library of Congress Cataloging-in-Publication Data
Hazard, David.
    Relieving headaches and migraines / David Hazard.
        p. cm. — (Healthy body, healthy soul series)
    ISBN 0-7369-0485-9
        1. Headache—Popular works. 2. Headache—Alternative treatment. 3. Naturopathy. I. Title.
    II. Series.

RC392 .H394 2002
616.8'491—dc21   2001051787

Printed in the United States of America.

02 03 04 05 06 07 08 09 / BP-VS / 10 9 8 7 6 5 4 3 2 1

Contents

Books by David Hazard
in the Healthy Body, Healthy Soul Series

Reducing Stress
Breaking Free from Depression
Building Cancer Resistance
Relieving Headaches and Migraines
Controlling PMS
Managing Your Allergies

Healthy Body, Healthy Soul

Common headaches and migraines are very different experiences, for sure. To the sufferer, however, the results can be the same: a painful disruption in the flow of life's work and play. For many, the reaction is simply to take a pill or a prescribed drug and hope for the best. And although these remedies can be useful, there are other ways—natural ways—that can bring relief from headache or migraine pain, or even prevent their arrival before they begin.

All of us, at one time or another, have experienced the common headache. But few of us understand how headaches begin. Generally, these intrusions into our routine are triggered by muscle tension. Stressed muscle tissue clenches tight on nerves and blood vessels, which radiates pain through the small muscles of the neck and head. This muscle tightness usually comes from stress in one form or another—from overworked or strained muscles, from blood vessels tensing to handle a sudden increase or decrease in pressure, or from chemical or hormonal changes and imbalances. It can even come from nonphysical sources such as mental or emotional pressures. These interior stresses can cause us, without knowing it, to tense our muscles. The result is as if our nerves and blood vessels have become painfully clamped in a vise.

Over-the-counter pain relievers can help relax this tension by slightly increasing the size of veins. This helps relax our muscles, releasing those squeezed nerves, increasing blood and oxygen flow again.

As for migraines—their origin is largely unknown as yet. In fact, there seem to be different types of triggers. Some migraine headaches may come from muscle tension and increased or decreased blood flow, specifically, to the brain. This kind of migraine is often helped by stronger drugs, available only by prescription, which help regulate blood flow and blood pressure. Other migraines are eased only by the use of drugs that block nerve impulses. This suggests that the trigger may be a chemical change within the brain's electrical system—because the sufferer sees, hears, smells, tastes, or feels sensations or emotions that have no known source.

Studies have shown that headaches and migraines can also be caused by a range of "hidden triggers," including:

- *intolerance to certain foods and food additives*
- *strain caused by wrong posture*
- *eyestrain*
- *emotional stressors*
- *spiritual tensions*

Though there appears to be, in fact, a wide range of headache and migraine triggers, recent studies in natural healthcare and natural medicines have begun to find that there are many simple and effective treatments for both. The very good news is that there are strategies you can do on your own to prevent, or to ease the pain of, common headaches and even migraines.

These natural approaches to headache and migraine relief are easy to learn. They begin with practical ways to find and resolve inner stresses that are often the trigger of physical tension. These include:

- *simple mind-relaxing techniques you can use anytime, anywhere, to ease the stress of mental and emotional overload*
- *personal spiritual practices that release the inner conflicts that can radiate into physical stress*

These natural approaches also include a wide range of things you can do to short-circuit physiological triggers of headaches and migraines, such as:

- *easy-to-make changes in your diet and eating habits*
- *herbs, vitamins, and other natural supplements*
- *a range of hands-on action steps—including headache-preventing exercises, massage tips, and personal acupressure techniques*

In this book, one of a series offering natural remedies to common health problems, you will discover many simple, natural remedies you can use to prevent and relieve headaches and migraines. And because the best treatment is a whole-person approach, you'll find that the wide range of strategies offered will treat the *whole you*—helping to restore health in body and soul.

David Hazard
Founder of The New Nature Institute

1

Easing the Pain

*D*o any of these statements about *headache pain* sound familiar?

- "I get headaches all the time. At least a couple times a week. Sometimes the pain relievers don't really help."

- "These constant headaches affect my ability to do what I want to do. They're also affecting my ability to enjoy life. How can I handle my responsibilities, or enjoy people, or have a good time when I'm nursing a headache?"

- "I am so tired of feeling headachy and wiped out. It's hard to be a good parent when my head aches and I'm crabbing at my kids or telling them to leave me alone."

Or maybe one of these statements—about those killer headaches known as *migraines*—better describes your personal experience.

- "I get migraines, and the pain is so horrible and intense it feels like my skull is being squeezed in a vise. I can barely handle it. My whole life stops. And even after the pain is over my mood is affected—I can feel irritable or depressed for some time."

- "The head pain is only part of it. All my strength goes, and I'm violently nauseous. One time I experienced hallucinations. Afterward, I'm kind of shaky and anxious for a day or two."

- "First come the 'auras.' I smell odors that aren't there. Or I
  see patterns before my eyes. Or I have the sense that something is just wrong—out of whack. Sometimes this develops
  into a migraine, sometimes it doesn't. Just the warning signs
  paralyze me. I don't want to go anyplace or do anything
  because *what if*...? What if I'm out somewhere and it *does*
  turn into a migraine?"

"I've Given Up Too Much Ground to Headache Pain...."

Whether you suffer from chronic or severe headaches of the
more common sort, or you experience the agony and debilitating
distress of migraines, you have probably come to the conclusion
voiced by this longtime sufferer:

"I woke up one day to the fact that headaches were limiting my
ability to work, love, have fun—to live. I had to plan my life around
my headaches, wondering when the next one would hit. Wondering
if the pain relievers would work or not—because sometimes they
just didn't. Also wondering if all the medications I was running
through my stomach might be harming me. When I read the possible side effects it was scary.

"I realized I've given up way too much ground to headache
pain. And I decided I had to find out if there was something I could
do—besides swallowing extra-strength pain relievers—that can
prevent them. Or keep them from becoming so severe. Or help me
get over them quicker when they hit.

"I wondered—are there good, natural alternatives that can ease
this awful pain?"

Whether you are a headache or migraine sufferer, the answer
is *yes*.

Take the Natural Approach—and You're in Charge

This book will help you learn dozens of these natural healthcare strategies, widely used by both traditional and natural healthcare practitioners alike. It will help you learn how to prevent, and
to ease, the life-limiting pain of headaches and migraines and live
well again.

R

IF YOU HAVE NOT SEEN A DOCTOR

∿

Headaches and migraines can be related to many under-lying health problems that only medical testing can reveal. If this is the case, it's best to detect these problems as early as possible. This gives you the best chance to successfully treat the problem and return to good health.

If you've been putting off a visit to the doctor…stop right now and make that phone call to schedule an appointment. You may benefit from medical testing, which can detect whether your headaches are caused by a more serious, under-lying problem—or free you of that worry so you can go on to find the right treatment for you.

Maybe you've already seen a doctor who has pronounced you "well." You may be wondering if he or she missed some-thing, or if they paid careful enough attention to the symp-toms you described. If this is the case, schedule a visit with a new physician.

If you are a migraine sufferer, you and your doctor may wish to establish a working relationship with a local emer-gency room or health clinic. Sometimes a migraine will only give way to strong medication introduced by injection. This can be done by emergency room or clinic personnel when you're in the grip of a migraine and your physician isn't immediately available to help you.

Although this book is a guide to practical, natural strategies you can use on your own, we emphasize that it's important to build good working relationships with a range of healthcare professionals.

If you're suffering from chronic headaches or from migraines, you will benefit from the care and guidance of people who are trained in the treatment of these painful maladies. Not all tradi-tional or complementary caregivers have the know-how. So as you look for the right people to help you, keep these things in mind:

- **No single professional can be experienced in all human ail-ments.** You will benefit greatly if you make one or more knowledgeable professionals part of your "care team." In addition to a medical doctor, you may benefit from the advice of an allergist, nutritionist, chiropractor, psychological counselor, naturopath, or herbalist...among others.

- **Not all medical professionals are "up" on natural and complementary techniques, such as those described in this book.** Most medical schools are just now adding courses dedicated to the study of natural and complementary healthcare, so you may find some doctors do not support the use of these strategies. Some may even refuse to treat you unless you agree to use only the traditional methods, such as the use of strong painkillers and nerve blockers.

- **Most caregivers—even "specialists"—are likely to approach your problem through the "lens" of their particular training.** A nutritionist is likely to say your problem has its basis in what you're eating or not eating, a chiropractor is likely to look for musculoskeletal problems...etc. Very often our health problems—including headaches and migraines— can come from more than one source...and resolving them may require more than one kind of treatment.

Only some caregivers are trained, or have trained themselves, to look at you as a whole person. These are the ones who will look at you and your problem in the larger context, taking into account mental, emotional, and spiritual needs...as well as physical needs. If you find a caregiver like this, you've located a valuable member of your personal team.

Most important:

- **Although you can benefit from the knowledge of a "care team,"** *you* **are the team captain.** We experience the very best in personal healthcare when we assume bottom-line responsibility for making choices about our own health and well-being.

Fortunately, there is growing knowledge and acceptance of natural and complementary practices among the traditional healthcare community. As a result, these caregivers are building better working relationships with the traditional medical community.

It is *very* important that you take the lead on your own behalf. You are the one whose health and well-being are at stake. You can only win by taking charge of your personal health, balancing what only you can know—the facts about what goes on inside your body and soul—with the experience of traditional and natural healthcare givers.

Create the Strategy that Works for You!

Maybe you're tempted to think, "Gee, this sounds like work. Wouldn't it be easier just to take a pill, and get on with it?"

Headaches and migraines are bad enough in themselves. The pain alone can be very hard to put up with. New breakthrough medications are helping headache and migraine sufferers find quick relief.

But the fact is, no medication will help you discover what triggers your pain in the first place. That, you must do. Likewise, a medication will not *un*-do the broader consequences that have developed when you've suffered pain over a long period of time— the "ripple effect" of pain that can spread and slowly encompass your whole life. Because this ripple has spread so slowly, most of us don't even realize how much ground we've really given up.

If it seems easier to "just take a pill"…step back and take a look at the bigger picture and ask: How has chronic pain affected your whole life? For example:

Recurring pain usually has serious emotional and social consequences.

Consider the time you've spent alone nursing a sick headache. Have you been robbed of hours that would have been better spent enjoying friends and family? Have you found yourself depending too much on other people to do things for you that might trigger a migraine?

Headaches or migraines can cause you to suffer career and financial consequences.

Have you missed hours or whole days of work when you could have been advancing yourself in your career and improving your earning power?

Surely you have personal dreams...also a sense that you want to make a bigger contribution to the world.

Consider how many times you've said "no" to volunteering for a good cause, because you felt headachy and worn. Consider—honestly—whether your vision of your life has been narrowed down to the pursuit of ways to avoid a headache.

Consider that wonderful sense you could be experiencing much more often—the sheer enjoyment of being alive.

Are you giving up pastimes you love—such as creative pursuits or hobbies? Or sports or other outdoor activities?

Wouldn't you like to be pain free more of the time...just so you can laugh...or hold and be held by...or focus on meaningful conversations...with people you love?

Without realizing it we can allow headache or migraine pain...or even the *fear* of it...to impose real limits on the way we live. We suffer consequences far beyond just the physical pain.

We suffer from psychological consequences because we lose the excitement that comes from healthy, forward-looking possibility thinking, and we begin to feel stalled. We can even suffer in spirit—because whenever pain is chronic or severe, whenever life is limited, we may wonder where God is and why nothing is being done to ease our pain.

When we really stop to look at it, it's far more than "just" the headaches, isn't it? When we look at the bigger picture, we start to see why "just taking a pill" cannot stop the slow, quiet devastation that chronic pain can spread through our whole life. We have to take into account the collateral damage suffered, which can include: lost dreams and aspirations, social isolation, a sense of purposelessness, depression, hopelessness...and a sense that our whole life may be passing us by.

Take Back Your Life—with a "Whole-Person" Approach to Wellness

Maybe you've tried over-the-counter medications or even strong pharmaceuticals to relieve your suffering—that is, you've tried the best that traditional, modern medicine has to offer. Quite likely, such medications have given you some relief. For that reason,

I am not advocating that you stop using these medications at all to help ease your pain.

Nonetheless, there are also many natural strategies that address your health needs as a whole person—things you can do *without* the help of a doctor or drugs. For, as many doctors will tell you, just taking a pill will not help you discover the causes that trigger your headaches. That's something you must do, and this book will help you. Nor will pharmaceuticals help you recover ground you've given up. That's also part of your task...and, again, the techniques you'll find in this book will give you a great new beginning. Because as you find your pain triggers—and there is likely to be more than one trigger—you'll find that you can make healthful changes that ease your suffering *and* give you back your whole life again.

As millions of everyday people and healthcare professionals are discovering, a *whole-life* approach to easing pain and curing illness is *the* most beneficial approach. If you want...

→ **effective pain relief techniques**

→ **new energy for living**

→ **and a whole-life sense of well-being**

... you've come to the right place!

Find Relief from Pain...Today

What follows are dozens of practical strategies. Many involve simple changes and techniques you can try today...and use anytime, anywhere. Other strategies you'll want to work into your life over time, to help you build healthy new habits that can keep you headache- and migraine-free.

In the next chapter we'll learn the first set of strategies—those that will help you relieve the most common trigger of headache and migraine pain: *mental stress.*

Whether you're looking for immediate relief or for long-term solutions, what you're about to learn will help you ease the pain of headaches and migraines...*naturally.*

2

"Tracking" Your Headache

You feel the pain coming on. You reach for a pill, or you lie down and apply a cold compress to your forehead. The problem is, sometimes this works...and sometimes it doesn't. Have you ever stopped to consider why this is so?

Most often a headache is really only a symptom of something else that's going wrong in your body. A muscle in spasm, pinching a nerve. A reaction to some allergen or environmental toxin. Body chemistry thrown out of balance by food that's disagreeable to you, or by an additive. Though we focus on the obvious pain, the fact is, that pain is being triggered by some other factor.

Unfortunately, most of us are "too busy" scrambling to cover all the bases in our demanding, everyday lives to stop and notice important details—maybe like the fact that we often have a migraine just before a trip home to see Mom or Dad, or two hours after drinking a glass of wine. As a result, the thing that can trigger our headaches remains unknown to us.

Instead, most of us have chosen the course of quick relief. Maybe we've been told that it's impossible to find the source of our problem because the body and the nervous system are "just too complex." So we've trained ourselves to pop a pill—whether that's an over-the-counter or prescription pain reliever. On one hand— why not? If we can get rid of pain fast with minimal effort, what's wrong with that?

But if we're truthful, we have to stop and ask—What *kind* of relief are we really getting? And what are these pills doing to our body?

If we could track down the things that trigger our headaches and migraines and resolve those problems—and do it naturally, without drugs—wouldn't that be a better solution?

Today more and more people who have resorted to the "just give me a pill" approach are agreeing that derailing headache pain at its source would indeed be a better option. In fact, a large percentage of headache sufferers report that the real results of pill reliance are not that satisfying:

- "At best, the pain relievers I take will knock the edge off a migraine. But I still can feel a dull ache."

- "Even if I take these [pills] with food, I get a burning feeling in my stomach. Or I feel a little nauseous."

- "I'm concerned that I'm becoming 'addicted' mentally, if not physically, to these pain relievers. I rely on them way too much, and I don't like that. When I realized I was taking them every morning to keep from getting a headache, I thought, *This can't be good for me.* Then I read a report about what pain-relief medications do to your stomach over time…*Wow.*"

- "Some days I take six extra-strength pain-relief capsules. In a really bad period I've taken as many as *nine to twelve* in a 24-hour period. That makes me very uneasy because I know that's not good for my body."

- "What concerns me is that in about three or four hours, when the medication wears off, the pain comes back. So what good are these pills *really* doing, if they're just masking the problem?"

- "I'm afraid of the kickback that's coming when these [pain relievers] lose their effectiveness and no longer ease the pain."

Even if you are not that reliant on pain relievers—do you know what triggers your headache or migraine pain? Shouldn't you?

Getting to the Source

Every headache or migraine has at least one trigger, and often there is more than one.

Finding what triggers our pain requires us to pay attention to what's going on in our life. Becoming mindful of how we're living can help us recognize very simple triggers—such as foods that bring on headaches—and deeply ingrained life habits—such as relationships that cause stress and physical tension. For many of us, paying real attention to ourselves is a new idea, and it may sound selfish or like too much work. On the other hand, we may already be aware that we have some life habits that are not the best…and we may not want to face them because we're afraid we won't be able to change them.

But here's the truth: Understanding and changing ourselves and our lives is *always* possible.

What we need is:

→ a new commitment to ourselves and to our wellness

→ patience in turning around health and life situations that did not come about overnight

→ a willingness to correct imbalances in our lives when we find them

If you're willing to make that kind of commitment to yourself, what follows in this chapter can become one of the most important tools for self-discovery, for moving toward overall wellness, and for the relief of your headache or migraine pain.

Often when we find the root cause of our pain, it's directly tied to something that's out of balance in our lives.

This brings us back to the need to pay close attention to our lives again. Most of us are used to rushing through life, not paying much attention to our real needs. Often we live by our *wants* instead. Then when we're sick or in pain we expect mom, or our spouse, or the doctor—*someone else*—to tell us what's wrong and fix us. Though you and I can benefit from outside expertise *to a point*, it's time to change your sense of who is ultimately responsible for your well-being.

The bottom line is—*you are.*

The simple truth is, most people who recover from debilitating health conditions—from headaches to cancer—are the ones who take responsibility for their own well-being. They are the ones who seek, and *keep on seeking*—accepting what works, rejecting what does not work—until they find the solution that works for them.

Taking responsibility for your well-being does not mean you "go it alone," because we all need the insight, advice, and team support of other knowledgeable people. What it does mean, though, is that you start listening very carefully to your life—that is, paying attention to your body's responses to what goes into it…paying attention to conditions where you live, sleep, and work…paying attention to the people in your life and the effects they have on you.

When we are experiencing chronic pain, we do well to direct this kind of focused attention to our whole lives. Why? Because sometimes the root causes of our headaches are directly tied to something that is out of balance in some aspect of our lives. At bare minimum, we do ourselves a favor when we track down the root causes, or triggers, of our headaches so we're better prepared with raw data when we seek help from healthcare practitioners.

Headache and Migraine Triggers

A Self-Test

What follows is a simple self-test, divided into seven parts. Though this is not meant to be used as a diagnostic tool for medical purposes, it can help you gain some insights into the causes of your condition. It can help you focus your attention across the broad spectrum of your life and detect some of the things that may be triggering your headaches or migraines.

The seven lists of possible triggers following are by no means an exhaustive list, though many of the main ones are suggested. By focusing on the broad range of life's activities, you're more likely to see how and why pain begins…perhaps triggered by sources you would not have considered before.

As you go through the sections, you may want to record your answers in the spaces provided or on a separate sheet of paper. By all means, whenever you discover a possible pain trigger, share that information with your healthcare provider. Each question is preceded by a brief introduction, which gives you a context for the question that follows. Take time to think through your responses.

1. Intense mental activity can trigger headaches or migraines in several ways.

First, the intensifying of brainwave activity can cause enough change or disruption in the brain's electrical activity that terrible pain is generated from inside the brain itself. (This can be accompanied by other sensations, such as smells, auras, or numbness.)

Second, intense mental activity can cause us—without knowing it—to tense the muscles covering the surface of the head and those in the neck and shoulders. Along with that, we breathe more shallowly…and sometimes even suppress our breathing as we struggle for a solution. The result is oxygen deprivation to already tense muscles…resulting in muscle spasms that pinch nerves running up the neck to the base of the skull, triggering pain in the fine muscles of the neck and head.

Finally, when we're involved in intense mental activity, we're often using, and overworking, our eyes. As a result, the ocular nerves become strained, sending out signals of distress in the form of…pain.

I experience a headache or migraine after periods of intense *mental activity* such as:

	Yes/No
→ reading	✓ ___
→ studying or homework	✓ ___
→ taking a test	___ ___
→ meetings	___ ___
→ a business negotiation	___ ___

Church, w m

→ organizing or running an event or activity ✓ __

→ a public presentation __ __

Watching T.V. light

2. Physical activity can create a range of possible headache and migraine triggers.

The most common are pinched nerves, resulting from the use of muscles normally inactive...or from overworking any muscle. Almost any activity can trigger a headache if it aggravates an old muscle-nerve injury, such as a pinched nerve in the upper back, shoulders, neck, or head.

Second, when we're engaged in physical activity we are increasing our muscles' need for oxygen. If we're not trained in proper breathing, increased physical activity leaves our tissues starved for oxygen, triggering spasms and pinched nerves.

Too, physical activity causes us to give off moisture in the form of sweat. Something as simple as a long walk on a sunny day can cause us to lose quite a bit of body fluid, until our electrolyte balance is thrown off, triggering that tired and headachy feeling.

Finally, there are certain activities we should do only under the optimum conditions. For instance...reading requires the right kind of light (and possibly eyewear) for our eyes to work well...typing requires the right posture so we don't strain our back or neck....

I experience a headache or migraine after periods of *physical activity* such as:

	Yes	No
→ exercise	__	__
→ reading	__	__
→ walking	__	__
→ driving	__	__
→ physical work—		
• light or moderate *(like house- or yardwork)*	__	__
• heavy *(like carpentry, moving furniture, digging)*	__	__
• at a desk or computer	__	__
→ sex	__	__

3. Many foods hold the potential to trigger headaches and migraines.

Almost any type of food can react negatively with our body's biochemistry, creating a sort of "toxicity" in our system that results in headache pain. We may do well with bland and spicy foods, for instance, but respond poorly to foods that are acidic.

Secondly, many people are unaware of allergies they have to certain foods, food types, or food additives. Food allergies can cause a number of disorders...including headaches and migraines. It is well known, for instance, that the sulfites in wine lay some people low, as does the monosodium glutamate in many oriental foods. And sodium can create blinding headaches in people prone to various high-blood-pressure disorders.

It is less commonly known that certain physical conditions—especially those in which the intestines are raw and ulcerated—contribute to headaches and migraines. It works like this: As your food passes from the stomach, it reaches the intestines. If you suffer from intestinal disorders—such as colitis or Crohn's Disease—larger-than-normal food particles can be absorbed into the bloodstream through your intestine's tiny perforations. It is believed that this creates a situation in your blood chemistry that can then trigger headache or migraine suffering.

I experience a headache or migraine within one to two hours of *eating:*

	Yes	No
→ food of almost any kind	✓	
→ spicy food	✓	
→ acidic food	✓	
→ sweets		
→ meat		
→ dairy products (milk, cheese, eggs)		
→ certain vegetables		

→ caffeinated drinks or foods (colas, chocolate) ___ ___

→ wine ___ ___

→ any alcoholic drink ___ ___

4. Medications and even supplements can assist our bodies with one healthy function—and at the same time react negatively in relation to another function.

Without going into the complicated biochemical reasons for this, we should be aware that many "helpful" substances we take can be involved in triggering headaches or migraines.

I often experience a headache or migraine after taking *medications* or *supplements*, particularly those I take for_____.

5. Certain people—this is not a joke—can trigger subtle, or not so subtle, reactions in your emotional-response system, leading to a headache or migraine.

Many times our reaction to another person is based on subtleties. Sometimes, our reactions don't make sense. Other people may find a certain person charming, witty, fun, smart, attractive, godly, winsome. We—for reasons we may or may not even know—feel threatened, overwhelmed, agitated, suspicious, or irritated by that same person.

At other times there is no question—we are really at odds with someone else: with their values, their personality, their treatment of us and other people, their views.

In either case, the tensions that exist in our relationships can have a major impact on our physiology. And the result may be a headache or migraine.

I experience a headache or migraine after an encounter with *certain people,* such as

Yes No

→ one or both parents ___ ___

→ other family member(s) *n. a.* ___ ___

➜ boss or supervisor   ___ ___

➜ spouse or partner   ___ ___

➜ children   ✓ ___

➜ co-worker(s)   ___ ___

➜ neighbor(s)   ___ ___

➜ religious leader(s)   ___ ___

➜ acquaintances   ___ ___

particularly _M . a , H, _____ .

6. Environmental factors may lie at the root of some headaches and migraines.

The factors may be allergens (plant- or animal-based) or chemicals (even those used in building materials, carpeting, fabrics, or dry cleaning). We can also be adversely affected by poor lighting or air quality.

I experience a headache or migraine after I have been in *certain places,* such as

                                    Yes No

➜ in my home, or the home of a friend   ___ ___

➜ in a certain room in my home   ___ ___

particularly _ma f c _____ .

➜ at work   ___ ___

➜ in outdoor settings   ___ ___

particularly _____ .

7. Change, in its many forms, has a much greater impact on our biorhythms than most of us know.

Think about the daily rise and fall of the ocean tides, and you get a rough idea of what biorhythm is to our total being. There is in each of us a subtle "rhythm" of life, and when it is disturbed, the ripple effects can throw off body chemistry, sleep, and eating habits.

We are all affected by such changing natural forces as the rhythms of *light and dark, seasonal weather shifts, traveling out of our time zone, long-distance moves, atmospheric changes in general,* among others. There are also certain biorhythmic hormonal changes we all experience. Though women are normally more aware of these rhythms than men, men experience them, too, both for biological and psychological reasons.

In any case, for various reasons, change can also trigger the onset of headaches and migraines. Sometimes, when a change is more of a long, slow progression than an overnight switch, it is harder to detect its relationship to the onset.

I experience headaches or migraines when there is *a change* in

	Yes	No
→ seasons	✓	
→ light	✓	
→ the weather	✓	
→ a relationship	✓	
→ work tasks or duties required of me		
→ my daily routines, personal habits, or schedule		
→ my sleeping patterns	✓	
→ my location or travel habits		

Armed with Self-Awareness

Hopefully—if you've taken time to go through these lists— you've made some discoveries. Or maybe thinking about the various aspects of your life and personal being has raised some questions for you.

If nothing else, this self-test—which you may want to repeat occasionally—can help you recognize the importance of developing your self-awareness. As one leading physician puts it, "It's amazing, and a little scary, how many adults cannot tell you what they ate for breakfast." Self-awareness—even a small amount of it—is crucial, whether you are seeking help from a professional or you are using the natural remedies such as the ones that fill the remainder of this book.

Now, armed with this new measure of self-awareness, let's look at the wide range of strategies you can use to ease headache and migraine pain naturally.

3

Mental Stress

Y ou've been feeling pretty good lately. Cruising along in life, pain free. Haven't been laid low by a headache or migraine in some time.

And then...you feel so good you volunteer to help with your kid's sports team. Or with a community or church activity. Or you sign up for the college course you've wanted to take.

In a short time the pain in your head is back.

Or maybe a set of pressures slides in like an avalanche....Bills stack up. You get involved in a grinding conflict with someone in your life. Your boss turns up the demands.

One morning you awake and it feels like someone has driven a metal spike through your temples.

Or your head just gets overloaded....The house and yard. The cars. The kids. Your work. Every aspect of your life, everyone in your life, is handing you a "To Do" list. And that handy little organizer you call a brain is trying to schedule time for all these responsibilities...but heading for a nuclear meltdown.

Mental stress is one of the most common sources of headaches and migraines. And it can be one of the most overlooked. We usually associate stress with physical tension because we can touch a tender or tense muscle and feel the results of overwork. But mental stress is just as taxing on our whole being, and the pain it generates is very real and debilitating.

Later in this book you'll find a chapter devoted to strategies you can use to ease physical tension out of your body. It's important to know how to prevent the muscle clenching that pinches nerves and sends a net of pain waves over your skull, and also how to ease physical tension once it's got you in its grip.

The strategies in this chapter will help you deal with a different, earlier set of pain triggers. Those that originate right between your ears, beginning as stress within your mind. Mental stress causes us to breathe shallowly, and to tighten our muscles the way we do when bracing for a collision. Most times we're so focused on our thoughts—anticipating a conflict, trying to figure out when and how we'll handle our crushing "To Do" list—that we don't notice how our stressed mind-set is affecting our bodies.

Instead of allowing mental stress to translate into physical tension...triggering more headache pain...you can learn simple techniques to stop this chain reaction from happening.

Here are some of the most effective, mental-stress relief strategies you can use.

Strategy #1: "Open the Door...Step Outside"

Ever notice what happens to your body when you focus on a problem, a task...or a long "To Do" list?

As mentioned previously, our breathing gets shallow and our muscles tense. The energy of our whole being starts to bear down on the thing that's holding our *zeroed-in* concentration. Our goal is to get this task done and out of our way! Even our eyes focus in, creating tension in the ocular nerves and throughout the small muscles of the neck, face, and head. We might picture what's going on like this:

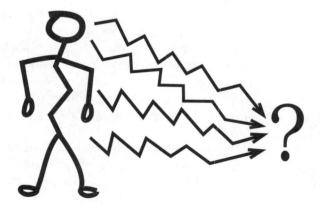

This kind of intensity can create both mental and physical stress…a leading trigger of headache pain.

One of the simplest things we can do to release the pressure is to "open the door" of our own intense concentration and "step outside" of it for a moment. We do this to expand our focus, which lets the pressure out of our body, in turn allowing our eyes and muscles to relax. We might picture this kind of open, expansive, relaxed focus this way:

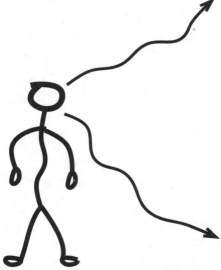

Opening our focus, which triggers the relaxation response, is the kind of thing we often do naturally when we walk outside and let our eyes focus on some distant point—the hills, the sky, a tree far off in a field. Hence, the name of this strategy.

Whether you choose to literally "open the door and step outside" or practice this strategy indoors is up to you.

Do This:

Step One: The next time you are caught up in a task that's forcing your attention into tight focus…stop and let yourself become aware of the tension in your body. Feel how it affects your eyes, your muscles, your breathing.

Step Two: Gently lift your eyes...and let them focus in the distance. (Obviously, this is easier if you're at a window or outside.) Your gaze will naturally tend to drift up and come to rest. Mental/visual relaxation is being restored.

Step Three: The natural relaxation this triggers will likely cause you to take in a deep, cleansing breath. Or you may yawn. This is because your body is expelling carbon dioxide that's collected in your blood and lungs. Do it again!

Let your breathing fall into a natural rhythm...which will usually be like a wave pattern.... A few normal or shallow breaths...followed by a deeper cleansing breath. Physical/emotional relaxation is being restored.

You can use this strategy to release mental stress even at school or at work. In case you're worried that it may break your train of concentration and derail your efforts—have no fear. It will actually help you return to your task with increased focus...and a much better frame of mind.

Strategy #2: Letting "It All" Go

Some of us are "stress batteries." Every care, every pressure, every responsibility turns into worry energy. Not only do we carry our own problems deep inside, we pick up concerns from other people. As a result we live in a state of tension and subtle anxiety.

When we're tense our whole physiology is affected. We don't breathe deeply and freely, so our muscles become oxygen deprived. We also send signals throughout our nervous system that say, "Brace for a crash"—again, tensing our muscles.

Along with this negative stress energy, some of us are also plagued by very distinct *intrusive thoughts*. These may come in the form of stress-inducing statements. ("You're going to lose...your job...your health...everything.") Or your intrusive thoughts might come in pictures. These may be of a general nature—such as a "towering wall" or "a cage" of pressuring responsibilities. Or they may be mental pictures of the thing you're afraid of—such as losing a person you love or being confronted by someone/something that will harm you.

We need to learn how to let go of our cares, worries, and anxieties. We're not talking about *bailing out* on genuine responsibilities. We're talking about learning how to *relax into* a new sense of inner calm. As we do this, we set aside our cares long enough to give our body, mind, and spirit a needed break, and this short-circuits the tension that triggers pain.

Do This:

Step One: Sit in a quiet place where you will not be distracted.

Step Two: Focus on your breath. Breathe in slowly and deeply through your nose, allowing your diaphragm to expand. Let the air out gently through your mouth.

As you continue to focus on the tide of air flowing in and out, allow your breathing to take on a natural rhythm. Feel the tension drain from your being with each breath you expel.

For many people, these two steps alone are enough to trigger deep relaxation. But if you're plagued by intrusive thoughts, you may benefit by adding this additional step:

Step Three: Let the mental stress you feel create a picture in your mind. Some describe their sense of being overwhelmed by tension like this: "I feel like I'm trapped in a room without doors, and it's filling up with water." Or, "I'm surrounded by high walls on all sides...and they're collapsing in on me, and I'm going to be crushed."

If your imagination is involved in creating mental stress:

- Continue the relaxation breathing. Don't fight the stress-inducing image—allow it to arise very clearly in your mind.

- In your mind's eye, let a hole or opening appear in the "wall" that surrounds you. With each breath you exhale, "see" the pressure rush out...or "see" yourself stepping through the wall completely calm and unharmed.

- Or...imagine the terrible event you fear coming right to its worst point...but this time watch as some other "force" intervenes. As you watch the tragic scene "freeze frame," consider all the forces in this world that *can* intervene on your behalf....Police or rescue workers...clergy...friends or family ...even God. Picture the tragedy being diverted with the help of one or more of these forces...and imagine the scene unfolding with a good outcome instead.

℞

ANXIETY DISORDERS

～

Some people literally cannot stop the intrusive, distressing images or voices in their heads. They're plagued with a sense of inner distress, sometimes close to panic, and feel themselves to be drowning in the pressure of anxiety. This may signal that they are suffering from an *anxiety disorder*.

Though you should not attempt to diagnose yourself or anyone else, you should also know that anxiety disorders are on the rise. They are thought to result from a problem in brain chemistry—in particular, an imbalance in the neurotransmitter chemical *serotonin*.

Anxiety disorders will make you feel compelled, or pressured, to do certain things in an attempt to escape the intense anxiety you feel: intrusive thoughts and images..."crazy" thoughts that you know are untrue...ritual counting...ritual touching...grimacing or blinking...difficulty eating or keeping food down...a body image that does not match reality...washing and rewashing...a fear of contamination...compulsive neatness that borders on mania—these can all be signs that an anxiety disorder is present.

If you suspect that you or someone you know is suffering from an anxiety disorder, consult a physician, psychologist, or psychiatrist immediately.

Those who practice this strategy will experience immediate and positive benefits.

First, focusing on our breath directs our mind away from stress-producing thoughts. This, along with the act of breathing more deeply, triggers the "deep relaxation response" that is an important foundation to physical well-being.

Second, letting out stress along with our breath literally keeps stress in its place—which is outside of us! The sense of being overwhelmed diminishes as we actually feel stress's negative energy shrinking down to a size we can manage. In place of fear or panic, our emotions come back into our control.

Finally, by learning how to stop and look at our stresses from a different angle, we take a step toward a more balanced and mature perspective. Life does have its stressors...but they don't have to control us. We can direct them instead.

Strategy #3: Check Your "Reality Filters"

Much of our mental stress comes from the way we are trained to think about things. Every one of us has a sort of mental "filter" through which we look at the world.

Some of us head out the door every day thinking, "The world is a crummy place. No one cares about anyone." Or, "I wonder what bad thing is going to happen to me today?" Or, "If something rotten is going to happen, it's going to happen to *me*." Or, "How do I know if I'll make it back home in one piece?"

In short, our view of life and the world is very negative...and this negative filter through which we view reality creates a negative inner climate.

It's true that life has lots of challenges—and sometimes we get more than our fair share dumped on us. But there's a difference in agreeing with the realistic voice inside that says, "The world can be a tough place, and difficult things are going to happen to you sometimes; be prepared," and listening to the cynical voice that says, "This whole world is rigged to go against you, and the worst is going to happen to you...and probably sooner than you think."

A negative mind-set is one very powerful source of mental tension. Sometimes we're aware of it, sometimes not. When it exists, it can be an almost constant trigger for physical tension.

We need to fight against a negative mind-set—including the idea that we're destined for misfortune—the way a nation fights against an invading army. *That's exactly what it is.* We need to resist it, both for the sake of our mental well-being and because it exerts an incredible amount of interior stress.

What can you do to remedy a negative mind-set that induces stress?

Granted, a mind-set forms over a period of time, and it can take time to reverse that old habit of negative thinking. But these steps will help you begin turning things around.

Do This:

Step One: Wait until the next time you catch yourself thinking negatively…or intentionally call to mind negative things about life that leave you stressed. Perhaps you carry around mental images of the way friends "always" let you down. Or the way your boss or co-workers *never* reward or even notice your hard work. Or you carry a bank of memories of the times your chronic headaches, or something else, have prevented you from enjoying life.

In your mind's eye, "freeze frame" the scene.

Step Two: Evaluate what you are telling yourself as you envision what your life is like. This helps you locate and identify your "inner interpreter." This is the voice inside that tells you what to think about what you're experiencing, and it has a definite attitude.

As you listen to your own commentary about your circumstances, ask yourself these three questions:

- What is this inner voice telling me about my *unpleasant experiences?* ("You have so *many* bad things happen to you. More than all those *lucky* people.")

- What is it telling me about *life in general?* ("Life is tough, and then you die." "Life is just trouble and suffering." "Life is not fair.")

- What is this voice telling me about *me?* ("You deserve this…" [or] "You don't deserve this…but you don't have the power to do anything about it.")

Step Three: Challenge your "inner interpreter." When your mind-set is on the negative side, your view of reality—the filter through which you see things—needs to be set right. So…

- Challenge…statements that magnify the scope of your unpleasant circumstances. ("It's not true that *everything* in my life is bad. There are good things in my life, and I'm going to focus on them right now, to bring the picture into balance.")

- Challenge…statements that color "the whole world" or your "whole life" in somber, unpleasant tones. ("It's not true that the world is totally… *unsafe… unkind… uncaring… unfriendly …unrewarding* of all my best efforts. Sometimes I win, sometimes I lose. Sometimes bad things happen to me, sometimes good things happen. We all have good times and bad times.")

- Challenge…statements that put you down. ("I am not a loser. I am not a 'problem-on-two-legs.'")

Step Four: Re-educate your interpreter. Expose him/her to different perspectives that take a more balanced view of reality.

- "The truth is, tough things happen to everybody. Everyone has something difficult or unpleasant or painful to deal with at some point in their life."

- "Life is not all bad. The world is not just scary or challenging. It's also full of good. I am going to look at life, and view the world, in a more balanced way."

- "When I keep a balanced view of life and living, I am taking the mature, adult view of reality. Then no matter what circumstances I find myself in, I'm the winner. Winners know how to take the good with the bad."

Strategy #4: Create "Head Space"

Someone has figured out that we only use about 10 percent of our brain's capabilities. This discovery seems to have become fodder for the current motivational rhetoric that says we "owe it to ourselves to achieve our full potential." Do we ever stop to notice who it is that pushes this line the hardest, or ask ourselves what their motive might be? Usually, it's sales and marketing managers chasing a big bonus, or New Age gurus selling books and products, or the preachers of "positive thinking" building a following. Sometimes it's parents who want to realize *their* unmet dreams through their children. ("I never made it, but *you're* going to.") In short—people who often have a personal interest in having us achieve.

On the other hand, some of us just naturally overload our schedules. We believe it's our job to do as much as possible to keep everyone…safe, happy, healthy, fed, provided for, and/or entertained. We feel guilty if we don't sign up to help with every cause. And along with that, we're concerned about what our neighbors might think if our lawn and garden looks a little less manicured and our cars sit in the driveway unwaxed. ("Some of us were wondering if you're not feeling well…with your place going to the dogs like it is.")

It's time to stop pushing ourselves. Never mind guilt and obligation. Forget the neighbors.

The mind can become overloaded and overworked. Sometimes we simply need to empty our heads of all the stressing details, plans, and schedules that badger us for attention. We need to get rid of nonessential worries…all those tensions we actually create for ourselves.

We need time and space just to *be*.

Do This:

Step One: Purchase a small pad or notebook and make a list of the various projects and duties for which you're responsible. Sometimes just the act of making a list, rather than carrying details around in your head, releases a significant amount of mental stress.

Step Two: Look at each project and ask yourself, "Am I the only one who can do this task, or can someone else do it?"

Some of us are natural doers. Because we *can* handle a task, we think we *should* do it.

Some people take on the tasks that other people should be doing. We think and act for everyone. We may believe we're doing them a favor, but we're not. What we're really doing is turning ourselves into slaves and overloading our mental circuits (our physical and spiritual circuits, too).

Oftentimes we just plain get overloaded and need help. When this happens we need to follow through and *get* that help.

Go down your list of responsibilities and:

→ **reassign** a task if it belongs to someone else and you're doing it

→ **prioritize** by being really honest about the tasks you care about...and those you don't

→ **drop** the tasks that are non-essential

Just as important:

→ **love**...or at least like, *half* of the tasks on your prioritized list...even more, if you can pull it off

Does this last part sound unrealistic? Then you need to work on this exercise more than you know. Far too many of us dislike the tasks we've taken on. That can be a sign that we're accepting too many of them out of obligation or guilt, at the same time allowing the activities we really do like to be squeezed out. (Could there be a connection between this and the unpleasant pressure that squeezes our heads? Yes!)

As you try this strategy, you'll be amazed at how much mental stress is released. You'll also be amazed how much your life changes. Few things relieve mental stress *and* add spark to life like allowing time for the pursuits we really enjoy and care about. Why do we need to create "head space"? Not only to clear out details and duties that are overstressing us, but to make room for the things in life that make our time here enjoyable.

Strategy #5: Talk Out the Tension

Often we carry within us the tension of conflicts we genuinely don't know how to resolve. We go over and over the conflicts in our heads, but never move toward a real solution. We can experience frustration...even rage...all in the form of an angry tornado of words trapped inside our head. The mental and physical stress this generates does very bad things to our whole being, and it wastes time that would be better spent living well.

If you don't have the option of walking away from the person or situation with whom you're in conflict, you have to work out your inner tensions. Mainly this will involve talking things out.

The problem for many of us, though, is that the words we need to say can get stuck inside.

Maybe we don't want to hurt another person's feelings. We're afraid our pent-up anger will be destructive when we let it out. Or maybe we don't like the discomfort *we* feel when we're in a conflict setting. We may tell ourselves we're being a "better person" for carrying the brunt of conflict.

To make it more difficult, some of us may come from backgrounds where we were taught to believe that "overlooking" or "accepting" difficult reality, conflict, and others' flaws means we are being "nice" or even "more spiritual." But our passive responses do not make the conflict go away, nor do they make us "nice" or "spiritual." They just make us more...well...passive. Also more overrun and more full of mental stress. Eventually, the stress becomes sickness or physical pain.

Do This:

Step One: Identify a conflict that is ongoing in your life. In a notebook, write down what the conflict is about—for instance, two values that are clashing or a disagreement about the facts of a situation. This will focus you on the core of the conflict, not the other party involved.

Step Two: Talk confidentially to a friend or counselor first. Tell them not only the circumstances...tell them what the core of the conflict is. Many times we talk to people just to unload our frustrations. Once the energy of our anger is spent, that's that. Letting off steam has some value—but not as much as coming up with a plan for working through the conflict.

Together, talk through an action plan.

Step Three: Create an action plan. This might include:

- *Determine your "terms" for a truce.* Sometimes we're not clear about what we're asking for—so how can the other person know how to respond? What *exactly* do you want the other party to do, to help resolve the matter in conflict? Which terms are absolutely essential for you to feel the matter is more or less resolved? Which ones are less important? (Meaning, you can be prepared to compromise on these points without feeling like you're losing.)

- *Write a script for yourself.* Some of us are not quick on our feet when it comes to thinking and dialoguing in a conflict situation. We lose focus. The other person swamps us with their logic. Or the atmosphere gets charged with emotion. We cannot direct what the other person is going to say, of course. But we do ourselves a huge favor if we know the points we need to make to represent ourselves well.

  There are many benefits to thinking through a script. It's like having a conversational map. We know where we need to go, what points we need to cover. This helps us recognize when the conversation is getting off on a tangent and helps us get it back on course. It also helps us maintain our cool, because we tend to tense up when we feel like we're losing our way in a difficult conversation, and tension triggers not only emotional outbursts but headache pain as well.

- *Know your "bottom line." State it clearly. Be willing to stick to it.* Sometimes indecision is a big problem. We're not sure where our own limits are. Or we say, "I refuse to put up with _____ any longer," or "I need you to _____"—but we cave in to resistance. Once we've stated our position, we need to *hold* our position.

- *Be ready to take action...no matter what.* Just having the conversation may not resolve our problem. When we approach a conflict we always face three possible outcomes—win, lose, or a tie. We have to be prepared for all three.

  Of course we must be ready to accept a peace agreement and thank the other person for working with us to resolve the issue. But we also need to be clear within ourselves about our actions if things do not work themselves out. This means having a plan and knowing exactly what our next step will be if the other person will not bend, or tries to stalemate things by stalling.

Resolving conflict begins with talk...but it must end in *action*. Real change. This is the way we build a healthy life. And it helps us make forward movement when conflicts bog us down and create mental stress.

R̶ SOMETHING LIGHT

∿

Most of us carry around heads that are full of duties and heavy with the weight of our responsibilities. Often our only relief comes at the end of the day when we flop down in front of the TV and watch some mindless program.

We would do ourselves good if we learned to enjoy "something light"—a small treat that lifts the weight off the mind—at several different times during the day. We can get this by tucking into our briefcase, purse, or desk:

- a book of humor

- a volume of poetry

- an inspirational book

There is nothing quite like...the sound and feel of our own laughter, the beauty of a well-turned phrase, or words that lift our mind above the ever-present grit of life...to restore a touch of lightness to our thinking.

Strategy #6: Escaping Mind Traps

"What you eat, you are," goes the old saying.

We can amend that to: "What you *think*, you are."

Earlier we discussed a strategy for "clearing" a generally negative mental filter that darkens our view of life. This strategy is a variation on that, for those who get caught in emotionally charged thinking that creates stress and pressure.

Emotions are not "bad" in themselves. But we can get "stuck" in certain *dominant emotions.*

To get an idea of how this works: Picture your thoughts as a stream flowing through your head. The stream itself is neutral …clear…made up of simple observations of the world around us. Into this stream we pour our emotions…or maybe one particular emotion we tend to have most of the time.

If we're carrying inside us a great deal of sadness, for instance, our thought flow will be tinged with sadness. There we are cruising along, not much aware of our streaming thoughts…until something triggers sadness. Suddenly, we are very much aware. We are *sad.*

Without noticing it, a big shift in our attention takes place. We have shifted our focus from the outer world to the inner. We are caught up in noticing our own feeling, and the more we focus on it the more it intensifies. In minutes we're wondering, "How did a good day suddenly turn so gray?"

Most of us believe we have no power over what goes on inside us. We let ourselves be dragged down into the emotions that capture our attention. We are, effectively, caught in a mind trap.

What's happened is that our thought flow has developed an "eddy"—like one of those swirl patterns you see on the surface of a river. The flow isn't moving forward, it's going down.

We are caught up in painful, unhappy feelings. Logic, which helps us move through feelings by resolving them, may stop altogether. This is why it is a "mind trap," because the more we focus on the feeling, the more it intensifies…and the more mental stress we experience.

Let's be clear on this: Emotions are not "bad" in themselves. And sometimes we do need to stop and explore our emotions with the help of a professional counselor who will let us air our innermost thoughts and feelings so we can understand them. But the point of exploring unpleasant feelings is always to move on from them.

The good news is, we can escape mind traps and the mental stress they cause. Whether you are working with a counselor or working on your own, this strategy will help you.

Do This:

Step One: Pay attention to your "thought stream" for a day. Be prepared to notice when you get caught up in a "mind trap" that drags you down into an intense emotion.

In particular, watch for mind traps that are created by emotions such as:

- *jealous or resentful thoughts*
- *frustrated or angry thoughts*
- *a sense of rejection or abandonment*
- *fearful or anxious thoughts*
- *overfocus on discomfort, illness, or loss*
- *self-pitying thoughts*
- *competitiveness—comparison thinking, anxiety about "losing ground" to someone else*

Step Two: Recognize that you have some power at your disposal, and it can help you escape your own mind traps. Accept this power as one that is God-given.

Too often, we spend our lives lying to ourselves, saying, "He *made* me angry." "She *made* me sad." "That [old injury, or recurring ailment] gives me a headache and makes me avoid [other people, the outdoors, the life I really want to live]." "So it's *their* fault I'm feeling stuck."

When we blame other people or circumstances for the way we feel, we've given up our personal power. What power is that? *The power to direct our focus.*

Think about it. We alone have the power to choose the aspect of reality on which we'll focus. No one *makes* us focus on…the sad, the unfair, the aggravating…or on our losses and ailments. We are the ones who direct our mind's eye and make those choices.

The good news is, we can learn to make better choices about our life focus.

Step Three: Practice changing your focus.

The next time you notice your focus swirling down an unhappy emotion, intensifying your mental stress-level:

- Stop, take a deep breath, and focus on your breathing. Do this until you feel calmer and more able to make a choice about your thought content and what you want your focus to be.

- Don't bother trying to tell yourself, "The bad things in my life are really good for me." Or, "I shouldn't feel hurt or disappointed." Or, "I shouldn't chafe inside when I have to accept tough realities. Forget it. Bad is bad. Tough is tough."

- Do choose to pour into your thought stream positive or uplifting emotions that *balance* the unhappy, negative ones. For instance, if you often get trapped in the misery of resentful thoughts about the fact that you have chronic headaches that are painful and limit you...balance them with factual observations about what you accomplish and how good you feel when you *don't* have a headache limiting you.

- Continue to work at blending your thoughts about the tough and unpleasant side of reality...with observations about the good side of it until you experience peace and a better thought flow.

And while you're at it, you might ask yourself, "What have all my experiences in life—the bad and the good—taught me? To whom can I pass on this understanding, for their benefit?"

Life is much better when we learn how to move on and not be trapped by the unpleasant. When we learn how to free ourselves from mind traps we release a tremendous amount of unnecessary mental stress and the pressure it generates throughout our whole being.

Deeper Still

Deeper than our mind, there lies another level of our whole person. This is the part we refer to as our *spirit*. Much stress generates out from this core level of being, triggering tension and reactions throughout our body and resulting in a number of ailments including an aching head.

For that reason we'll turn now to spiritual strategies that can aid us, ultimately, in easing tension, headaches, and migraines.

4

Stress and Spirit

*D*eeper than our thoughts...and even deeper than our emotions...there is a level of being we know as the spirit. If we carry tension at this deepest level of our life, science is now discovering, we stress our whole being and open ourselves up to many ailments—from immune disorders, to cancer, to headaches and migraines.

Each religious tradition defines the spirit a bit differently. For the purposes of this book, we're referring to our spirit as the part of our being where we hold

- *our most important values*
- *our beliefs about ultimate realities*—including our beliefs about the meaning of life, about God, and the way we think we should treat other people

There is another element to our spirit, one that has tremendous power to cause us to experience deep calm and peace...or to cause us deep turmoil, anguish, and stress. I am referring to

- our *conscience*—that light of inner knowing with which we observe ourselves and gauge how we're *really* doing in relation to our values and beliefs

In terms of spiritual health, the phrase "in relation to" is very important. That's because we as humans have the odd capability of holding on dearly to values and beliefs in our head...and then living in opposition to what we value and believe...and often, we don't notice the huge gap.

It's this problem—living in tension with our greatest values and beliefs—that causes deep-level spiritual stress in our lives. When stress exists in the core of our being, its shock waves will radiate through the rest of our being, even resulting in physical tensions and illnesses.

Consider these cases:

Howie

Howie's head-crushing migraines began within a year of taking over the family business. It wasn't exactly stress or workaholism. He had good support help and got plenty of sleep and exercise. The medications prescribed for his migraines harmed his stomach, so he sought other answers.

With the help of a counselor, he was able to put a finger on the source of a constant uneasiness that he could never escape. When he was just an employee, working in the family business was no big deal. But once he became head honcho, deeper issues came into play.

"All the weight of the whole family's future and well-being came down to *me*," he says. "If I failed, *everyone* failed. Not only was the whole success/failure thing going on inside me, I let it become a matter of my *worth*. I had to make the business even more successful...or at least not screw it up. At some really deep level my value as a human being got wrapped up in it."

At a spiritual level, Howie was living way out of balance in relation to reality. Though he was and is a good businessman, he had to realize that his worth as a human being is not measured by how much he grows the family business. And that he is not responsible for the success and happiness of his whole, extended family.

By using certain spiritual practices, Howie learned how to focus on his fundamental worth apart from his work. He began to gain from living more in sync with his spiritual values. In a few months he realized the intensity of his migraines was lessening. In time, they ceased altogether.

Cheryl

Cheryl's chronic headaches came on seasonally. Each winter, just after Christmas, they began and grew in severity for several months. At the worst point, she'd be popping extra-strength pain relievers all day for a few weeks. Suddenly, in late spring, her headaches would diminish, then stop altogether.

Allergies were discounted. Her hormone levels didn't seem to be a problem. At different times, she sought counseling for the strains that came from being a working mother, and also for some marriage tensions. But common stress didn't seem to be the trigger.

Nine years into this cycle, Cheryl experienced a renewal of her faith, which had lapsed when she was a teenager. It was while talking to her minister one day, discussing her journey of faith, that Cheryl ran into a blockage, or as she put it later, "In my spirit, it felt like I'd come up against a sort of 'locked door' I didn't want to open, because it led into a 'room' of my soul where I didn't want to go."

In college, Cheryl says, she and her mother "bashed heads" over the issue of her Mom's severe drinking problem. Growing up with an alcoholic mother had been tough, especially during the holidays when her mom's partying and drinking was off the charts. The year Christmas ended in disaster for her younger sister, Cheryl blew. She and her mother tore into each other.

"You don't like my drinking? Well maybe I drink because of you kids," her mother yelled, accusingly.

Cheryl felt a rage she'd never experienced, and shouted back— "*Drop dead, mother!*"

That winter she refused to return home or even to speak with her mother by phone. "I told myself she could fall over dead and I wouldn't care. She was a selfish alcoholic, in my book. I hoped she *would* die and stop making our lives miserable." Cheryl had no intention of forgiving her mother or even seeing her until she cleaned up her act.

The news came in late March, from an uncle who tracked her down by phone. "Your mother fell asleep at the wheel and ran into an oncoming truck. She's gone."

"When those words hit me," Cheryl says, "I thought, *You told your mother to drop dead—and now she's dead. Look what you did.*

"Later on I was able to tell myself mentally I wasn't to blame. Mom was driving drunk. But there was the fact that I'd judged her and hated her and never forgiven her....That went deep.

"I didn't kill my Mom, but my anger *did* kill our relationship. And because there was no way to mend it, I couldn't face that. I sort of 'closed the door' on the whole thing and walked away."

Walked away, that is, until she renewed her faith. Seeking a new, clear relationship with God, Cheryl wanted to be forgiven of her own past errors. And that's when she discovered the "locked door" to an inner room of the past, that "room" in her spirit which held her undealt-with anger and unforgiveness—and *remorse*—in relation to her mother.

From there, it didn't take a lot for Cheryl to make an important connection: The season in which she suffered chronic headaches every year occurred during roughly the same months as when the great tension and tragedy of her past took place. The link between the two seemed more than a stretch of the imagination.

"I really believe the headaches were symptoms of all the tension I carried—because as a daughter I wanted to forgive my mother, but I wouldn't let myself. Then this faith-renewal thing happened. The problem suddenly seemed obvious. Because it was too big a stretch for me to want forgiveness from God for my wrongs, when, even to that point, I hadn't forgiven my own mother for what her drinking did to us. In effect, I was saying to God, 'I want you to forgive me—but not *her*.' I could see the huge tension there."

Today, using Christian spiritual practices, Cheryl has been able to get a handle on the headaches. "I believe these strategies helped me face and deal with many different tensions that occur in my spirit. Last year," she reports, "I went through 'headache season' pain free. Also, I've generally been a lot healthier."

As these stories illustrate, there is a type of energy generated by the unresolved tensions that lie at the deepest levels of our being— and it's not a healthy energy. It's the negative, sickness-producing energy of stress, generated by the unfinished business of our spirit. That is, by old angers, longings, sorrows, unfulfilled hopes, and fears. By the unsettled "scores" of past violations against us...and the violations we've inflicted on other people. By the sense that we can't find our way. Both Howie's and Cheryl's stories illustrate how issues of the spirit cause deep-level tension, and how this stress sends continuing shock waves out through our whole being, negatively affecting us emotionally, mentally...and in time, physically...until it is resolved.

The Spiritual Strategies

There is not room here, and this is not the place, to discuss the basis or merits of Christian spiritual beliefs. What we'll focus on here are certain beneficial spiritual practices—sometimes called "spiritual disciplines"—which have developed in Christianity over the centuries.

These practices aid us in the business of living in a good, honest, and healthy relationship with our own spirit. Which is to say, they help us live in a healthy relationship with our core values and beliefs. Ultimately, if you are a believing person, you will recognize that they can help you live in healthy relationship with God and with other people—the two focal points of practical Christian spirituality for all time.

Regardless of where you stand in relation to Christianity as a faith, you can benefit from the spiritual practices recommended here because they work to release deep-level stress and support a healthy, balanced interior life. If you are not of the Christian faith, they may cause you to consider its claims...but we will leave that to forces outside this book.

Here then are six spiritual strategies you can use for deep-level stress relief.

Strategy #1: Quiet and Solitude

For most of us, life is filled with almost unending sound. We're buffeted by noise all day and tell ourselves we just want an evening of peace and quiet—which we then fill with TV or radio noise. For *maybe* a few minutes right before we fall asleep, we experience true silence.

If we're honest, some of us actually make sure our spaces of quiet and solitude are filled with sound. Truthfully, we don't *like* to be alone and quiet. Alone, we feel...*insignificant,* or *fearful,* or *guilty*...and these are uncomfortable feelings. Rather than face these feelings and undo the spiritual stress they cause, we hide in noise.

Yes, in silence and solitude we *do* face our innermost stresses. But when we face them and resolve them, inner balance is restored and we release the spiritual stress we've carried. And when we've achieved this deep-level relaxation our body is able to stop fighting against itself and return to health.

Do This:

1. **Set aside a specific time and place to be alone and quiet.** A few minutes a day is best. At minimum, make a space in your life for this weekly.

Choose a place where you will not be disturbed. This can be an out-of-the-way room in your home...or someplace away from home if you can manage it. The main thing is to be sure you're away from distractions like work, kids, the TV, and radio...and the phone.

You are looking for a place where you can experience stillness. Get comfortable.

2. **Do nothing...but focus on the stillness and quiet.** Doing nothing may be hard at first, because it means gearing down physically. Some of us are addicted, not only to noise and busy-ness, but to our own adrenaline.

Truthfully though, you are not here to do *exactly* nothing. You are here to focus on the stillness and quiet that lies behind the world's noise and frenetic energy...and your own.

3. **Let your whole life "go."** Most of us know what it feels like to have our whole life feel like a burden. Or at least to have some part of our life weigh us down.

This is the time and place to let go of the burden for a while. Sure, you may have to shoulder it again...but not in this space of time.

You may find it helpful to pray: "God, I surrender my whole life...and all my troubles and responsibilities...to you."

Try deep breathing while you do this...and feel the weight of life lift from your spirit.

4. Let new energy return. When we surrender our stress energy to God, we allow ourselves to experience inner rest. For now...for just this time...be free and at peace.

When your time at rest is ending, you may find it helpful to pray: "Go with me from this place. Let me take this peace with me...and fill me with the strength I need."

Many people who practice silence and solitude find it so freeing and empowering that they make it part of their daily routine. Some consider it as essential to their total well-being as eating, sleeping, or exercising.

Strategy #2: Prayer

Science is rediscovering what people of faith have known for centuries. Prayer has a healing potency. As you noticed, prayer was part of the first strategy—and we are going to explore it further here.

Prayer is, in fact, one of the most potent antidotes to stress-based illnesses and disorders...including headaches and migraines. In general, people who pray regularly tend to experience better health than those who seldom pray or don't pray at all.

Some of us are only familiar with the "rote" prayers we learned as a child. There are other ways to pray, of course. Here are two kinds of prayer you can use to great benefit:

Talking to God

Sometimes we're like "stress batteries," storing our thoughts, experiences, and emotions inside. Talking things out let's us process stress energy and release it. But we don't always have people around to talk *to*. Or maybe we just don't open up to others easily.

Many people experience the stress-releasing benefit of simply "talking to God."

Do This:

1. Begin each day by acknowledging that God is real and present with you. This simple acknowledgment can open up the possibility for ongoing talk throughout the day. If you forget to do this first thing in the morning, you can still acknowledge God's real presence wherever you are—on the job, out in public, at work around the house.

Whenever you acknowledge God, you are *basing* yourself in a reality that's bigger than the everyday circumstances you can see, hear, and touch. Some people call this *spiritual grounding,* or *centering.*

2. *The moment you become aware of stress, talk it out with God.* When stressful events come up...when stress-inducing people get in your face...they draw your whole focus. The boss wants something done *now.* The demanding child needs help *right now.* Your spouse wants to hammer on that important issue until it's *resolved once and for all.*

When this happens:

- touch base with your spiritual center by pausing for just a moment

- breathe in deeply, to fill your lungs with air and oxygenate the blood

- breathe out a short prayer ("God, keep me calm")...and release toxins that would otherwise build up in your lungs and further stress your body

If you find yourself needing to "vent" to God sometimes, it's okay. Sometimes that venting includes feeling frustrated with God when life is too difficult or chaotic. God is big enough to handle our cares and frustrations. Consider the Bible's open invitation to "cast all your anxiety" on God's shoulders.[1]

Listening to God

The other half of prayer is *listening.* Listening, as we know, is always harder than talking.

When we listen to God, we're not listening for a "voice" *per se.* We're mainly learning how to shut down all those inner voices that stream through our head, including our own.

In practice, listening to God requires us to reach a balance of inner stillness *and* inner alertness. Those who practice this type of

---

1. First Epistle of Peter 5:7

prayer—sometimes called *contemplative quiet*—say they never "hear" anything. Instead, they say they experience a kind of *deep knowing* that gives them a solid sense of confidence about their life, the choices they must make, and the directions in which they must go.

This inner state—one of unshakable confidence—is what we're after. Not only do we sometimes encounter rare insights in this state, but it also triggers the "relaxation response," which releases deep-level tension and fosters overall well-being.

Do This:

1. Get comfortable...and focus on your breathing. The goal is to refocus your mind away from the external world. For this reason, it's helpful to focus your mind on the stream of air as you breathe...in through the nose...out through the mouth.

Many beginners ask, "What should I expect? How do I know if anything good is happening?"

Don't expect a spiritual sideshow—with bursts of light or angels appearing.

Do expect a heightened awareness. *Do* expect to sense your mind and spirit "detaching" and drawing aside from the demands of your everyday world...and even from stresses going on inside you. *Do* expect a restful and clear sense of objectivity—as if you are standing aside peacefully observing your life, and what's going on outside you, and also what's going on *inside* you.

2. Gently turn aside all "inner voices" and all "images." It's likely that, before you reach this place of the restful observation, you'll be distracted by certain kinds of inner voices. Don't be discouraged, it's just your busy mind at work. You're likely to hear

- a censoring voice—telling you what you're doing is a waste of time and that you should be *doing* something

- a critical or accusing voice—pointing out your various flaws and faults

You can't turn these voices off by direct force. You can only do it indirectly by refocusing on your breathing...and letting them fade out.

You are also likely to hear

- **nagging voices**—reminding you about errands and tasks and duties you need to do

You can turn them off by keeping a pad and pencil at your side. Quickly jot down important things you *do* need to remember... then you can return to your inner business, knowing you won't forget them.

Some people are troubled by intrusive and unwelcome images. Again, you cannot "force" these out of your head. But you *can* indirectly get rid of them by gently refocusing your thoughts on "empty" images—say, the open sky.

3. Gently turn your thoughts to God. At this point, you are likely to experience a kind of inner detachment. You are becoming "the restful observer." That is, you may sense that you are "observing" yourself and your life...in a peaceful, non-emotional way...from "outside" yourself.

No, you are not leaving your body or stepping into some mystical realm. You are experiencing something like a "God's-eye" view of yourself and your life. Saints throughout the ages assure us this is normal. If you are a person of faith, you can accept that this may be one way God shares thoughts and views and wisdom with us...by allowing us to see things through eyes that are transformed by a "higher perspective."

And if you don't experience this kind of "transcendent" moment...no worry. You *will* experience a profound sense of rest. That in itself releases deep-level stress and restores inner equilibrium.

4. Continue in this "restful observer" mode as long as you can. Eventually, you'll naturally experience something that feels like "resurfacing"—that is, like coming up from under water.

Those who practice this strategy find they can use it to some benefit just about anywhere to keep interior stress from taking over—for instance, while stuck in traffic or in the midst of a grinding daily schedule.

Strategy #3: Keep a Spiritual Journal

If you kept a diary in your younger days, recording the fun and interesting things you did... *this* is not *that.*

A spiritual journal is one in which you can explore the big questions and themes of life—most especially the ones that are important to you personally. The idea is not to explore heady or theological/philosophical dilemmas. It's to grapple with the real issues of your life—like some of these:

- My past has been full of chaotic or painful events. If there is a good and loving God, how do I make sense of that?

- I have dreams and goals that I haven't realized. How can I begin to fulfill them?

- I'm at a crossroads in life, feeling a little lost or unsure. What's my direction for the future?

- Certain aspects of who I am—my personal identity—make me uncomfortable. What does God think of me?

A spiritual journal can also be a place where you write in a more "stream of consciousness" kind of "flow." Often this is done in combination with "Listening Prayer," described in the previous strategy. In that case, you are recording the "deeper knowings" that come to you in personal silence and solitude.

That's *what* you do. Here's how.

Do This:

1. Purchase an inexpensive journal. This can be one of those "empty books," or a spiral notebook, or a looseleaf binder. Some people journal on their computer.

2. Keep it in a locked, safe place. The main goal is to be as completely honest and open with your soul's contents as possible. This is hard to do if while you're writing you think, *What if someone reads this?*

If there is a possibility of someone reading your journal...or if you intend to read it to them...there is a huge chance you'll be less than completely open and honest. You're very likely to censor your thoughts, to clean them up and make them "acceptable." In which case, you've defeated the main purpose.

Plan to keep your journal in a locked file or drawer. Some people go so far as to have a pact with a friend or spouse so their private journals will be destroyed or edited in the event of their death.

3. Set a regular time to write. Set a writing goal. Regularity is the key to letting the contents of your spirit "flow" out on paper. And "free writing" until you have, say, two...or three...or four...pages full is a good way to keep the flow going.

4. Face your personal issues honestly. Don't pretend you're "doing okay" if you're not. The point is to keep yourself from getting "stuck" going over the same spiritual ground again and again, instead of moving on in spiritual growth. (*Hint:* If you hear yourself complaining about the same things *this* year that you complained about *last* year...or if you're nursing old grudges or wounds...*you're stuck*. And you need to be straightforward if you're ever going to help yourself move on.)

5. Periodically review what you've written. Choose a time, maybe at the end of every month or every season, when you reread what you wrote before. This gives you a chance to:

- **Detect problem thinking.** Sometimes we reread our thoughts and realize, *That doesn't make sense.* Or, *I made a mountain out of a molehill.* Or, *I was dishonest about that.* Or, *I wasn't willing to face the truth about that situation...but I see it now.*

- **Pick up self-defeating attitudes.**

Strategy #4: Check Your Inner Atmosphere

As you may have noticed, spiritual practices very quickly introduce us to what's really going on inside us. We can be amazed to find out how out of touch with our inner selves we've really been. (That's why the tension is there.)

One thing we discover about ourselves is that we tend to carry something like an "inner atmosphere." Think of it as "the dominant weather pattern" of your soul.

This is another way to talk about attitude. Are you inclined to be agitated and restless—and release lightning strikes of sarcasm or anger? Do you tend to be cold and aloof—indifferent, or prod others with criticism?

Our attitude can be affected by outward things, for sure. By people and circumstances. But it can also be affected by how we think about God. (*Why* **did** *God put so many crazy people in my life? Why* **are** *there so many obstacles in my path?*)

Many of us carry deep-level attitudes toward God that are negative. They can be so ingrained we don't even realize how toxic they are. Because they're negative and toxic they stress us at a core level—and from there they affect our mental, emotional, and physical well-being as well.

When you suspect your inner atmosphere needs checking—

Do This:

1. Catch yourself in a moment when you're in a negative frame of mind—especially if that "moment" has lasted for days. Take time to understand the attitude that's clouding your inner being. Check for things like:

___ guilt	___ sadness	___ shame
___ indifference	___ anger	___ fear
___ self-pity	___ jealousy	___ distrust
___ hopelessness	___ bitterness	___ hatred
___ vengefulness	___ stubbornness	___ resentment

It's not always easy to detect some of our inmost attitudes.

Rob sought help from a counselor, saying, "I'm always frustrated and angry. I feel agitated for days, and then I get these terrible headaches." But as their conversations progressed, a deeper attitude became clear.

Stuck in a career he hated, Rob felt hopeless about his life. When he saw happy, successful men he felt frustration and anger. Rob had to face an attitude more basic than his anger—that is, his sense that he was stuck in a career he hated. Underneath the anger, Rob felt hopeless.

It took Rob time to realize his problem and work through it. It may also require patience and some honest soul-searching on your part to fully recognize the attitudes that are forming the atmosphere inside you.

2. Be honest with God about the state of your spirit. Make the contents of your spirit part of your prayer dialogue. If we can't admit to God what we're really feeling, to whom *can* we admit it?

Being honest about ourselves is the first step toward integrating the negative energies that—transformed—drive us into a healthier, better response to life. Who better than God to help us do this?

3. Don't ask for the unhealthy attitude to be taken away...ask for a healthier attitude to "pair" it with.

Our attitudes determine our actions. In that sense they give us energy. Even negative attitudes can be good when we use them to move us away from what we *don't* want. But we also need to add healthy attitudes to help us move toward what we *do* want.

Rob realized hopelessness was an unhealthy attitude. On its own, it left him depressed and de-energized. Its only "good" was that it told him he really hated what he was doing.

With the help of his Christian counselor, Rob began to pray and ask for *hope*. This meant refocusing on things that would make his life more full and happy. Of course, his whole mood eventually lifted. On the career front, he was also more able to take practical steps to change his life.

Not too surprisingly, as all the interior pressure of hopelessness let go, Rob's headaches gradually left him.

Attitude plays a much greater role in our life and our health than most of us know. Consider joining the many people who make a "spiritual atmosphere check" an important part of their daily spiritual regimen.

Strategy #5: Check Your Beliefs About God

Sometimes our deepest attitude of all—the attitude we take toward God—can leave us with a case of chronic, deep-level stress.

What exactly *are* your beliefs about God? Not what your religion or denomination *tells* you to believe—what do *you* personally believe? We're talking about your real attitudes toward God. What we might call "working beliefs."

Does your working belief tell you that God is

___ present	___ absent	___ knowable
___ a mystery	___ caring	___ uncaring
___ punishing	___ pardoning	___ helping
___ indifferent	___ angry	___ peaceful
___ demanding	___ giving	___ welcoming
___ rejecting	___ loving	___ stern

When it comes down to it, spiritual beliefs require us to make a big leap, don't they? For many of us, it feels "safer" to stand on the side of doubt and even unbelief. We actually become practiced at ignoring our beliefs. The problem is, we're also left shouldering all the responsibilities and burdens of life on our own.

Belief in God—the "working" kind of belief we're suggesting here—*is* a spiritual practice. We are all going to experience spiritual struggle and doubt. But if you look at the checklist above and discover you have a relationship with God that's more negative than positive, you are likely to be carrying deep-level stress. And that's harmful not only to your spirit, but to your physical well-being, too.

Too many people carry a heavy or negative spirit for years and never take any steps to get out of the interior rut they're in.

Do This:

1. Locate the "growth edge" of your working beliefs about God. (This is where a spiritual journal comes in handy.) Write out what it is you *do* believe about God...and also your doubts, misgivings, or negative beliefs about God.

For instance, you may write: "I believe God is the Creator...but I don't think God is involved in our everyday life." Or, "I believed God was good and that God cared about me. But someone I loved very much got sick and God didn't answer my prayers. I just don't know what to believe about God now, or if I can trust again."

2. Accept each question as a "quest." Turn the things you honestly wonder about into questions. For instance, "I would like to know, God, if you are really involved in my everyday life. If so, how?" Or, "I really don't understand why you didn't answer my prayers, and why _____ was not healed. Can you give me wisdom to understand this? How can you be good and caring but ignore desperate prayers?"

Christian wisdom tells us we are welcome to "ask," "seek," and "knock"[2]—and to stick with it until our quest is met with an answer.

3. Emphasize what you do believe right now. Now that your "growth edge" is clear...flesh out the working beliefs you hold now.

For instance, "God is the Creator...and that means I was created by God. And even though things are difficult, I do believe my life is a gift to me from God." Or, "Even though some important prayers seem to go unanswered, I do experience God's goodness sometimes—especially when I look at my children [or friends, family, work] and they make me feel happy and blessed."

4. Express your gratitude. Sometimes we let our spirits become toxic by focusing on what we don't have, or what we believe God has failed to do for us. In short, we focus on the negative. Life has its downers, that's for sure. But are we stressing our spirits, and carrying more deep-level stress than is warranted, because we're ignoring the good...and majoring in the negative?

Try being thankful for what you do have. You may be amazed how spirit lifting this is.

5. Be willing to stay on the "faith journey"...even if answers are long in coming. The truth is, our whole life will be a journey of faith. We can sit down beside the path right now and refuse to keep seeking. Or we can have more courage than that, and keep moving.

---

2. Gospel of Matthew 7:7

You might consider praying:

> *God, I want to know you…not just in my head, but in the core of my being. Because you are God, I am going to ask you to make yourself known to me in ways that only you can do.*

(As a person of faith, I suggest you be ready for just about anything.)

The goal of this strategy is not *only* to help us find our spiritual "growth edge" but to get us stretching and growing stronger in spirit.

In a later chapter we'll look at working out some physical muscle knots that cause headaches. For now, think of this strategy as one that will help you find and work out the stiff, knotted muscles in your spirit that are keeping you from being healthier and more vital in spirit…and most likely in body, too.

Strategy #6: Confession

Confession *is* good for the soul. And the body, too. Something as mechanical as a lie detector proves that. When we're not being honest, our blood pressure spikes. The tension that's created between what our spirit knows to be true and what we're saying is true is amazingly powerful. So powerful, in fact, that shock-waves ripple through our being so strongly they can be measured by little electrodes taped to the skin.

So…what do you suppose happens when we carry around *lots* of hidden and uncomfortable facts about ourselves? The answer is: *We experience chronic deep-level tension.*

Confession is a spiritual practice that allows us to let go of the things that stress our spirits and plague our bodies with tension. Many people schedule regular times with a spiritual counselor, a minister, or a spiritual director. Some who are carrying more serious or complicated concerns find it beneficial to work with a licensed professional therapist to release these inner pressures.

℞

SPIRITUAL COMMUNITY

～

Many of us carry a lot of inner stress because we shoulder so much of life's load all alone. If you've been "out of circulation" for a while and not part of a spiritual community...consider getting involved in one. Without good spiritual relationships, we carry too much on our own.

Becoming part of a spiritual community has many healthy benefits. One of the greatest is that it gives us a way to unburden ourselves of our stresses by sharing them with other people.

Spiritual communities come in different forms—such as churches, prayer groups, or support groups. Most especially, look for a group that can offer some or all of the following:

- **A positive view of God.** Some who lead spiritual groups actually have a very negative view of God. Their attitudes of cynicism and sarcasm leak through. Find a group where the view of God is positive, and also health- and life-affirming.

- **Support for people with your particular need.** You need to be able to discuss your inner stresses with people who really understand, and who can offer encouragement and genuine concern.

- **A safe atmosphere.** That is, one that's confidential, where honest questions are welcomed, and where practical support is available when you need it.

Do This:

1. Set up an appointment with a spiritual counselor, minister, or spiritual director. If you're unsure how to find one, contact the diocesan office for your area, or a local church. County and state governments may also have listings for counselors in your area.

2. Make sure the terms of your relationship are clear. You are right to ask that everything you discuss be kept strictly confidential. You should also be clear that this is your time to speak openly, to get "off your chest" everything you need to bring up. Confessing is not the same thing as counseling.

3. Allow time for a relationship of openness and honesty to grow. Even if you feel the need to talk about the contents of your spirit, it's likely to take a few visits together before you feel ready to disclose your greatest secrets. Relax, and open up at your own pace.

4. Treat this as a sacred experience. You may wish to open and/or close your time by praying (to yourself or with the other person). This is highly recommended, so that you are conscious of confessing your inner stresses in the presence of God.

5. Accept grace and pardon through human vessels. There is something very powerful, even divine, that happens when we hear the words, "You are forgiven." Accept these words as true.

6. Leave what's in the past with God. Yes, you may wish to make restitution for something you've done wrong. But as for the guilt and stress that came with the offense…leave that behind.

LAUGH MORE

∼

A proverb from the Bible says, "A merry heart does good, *like* medicine…"[3]

Scientific studies also confirm that when we laugh, our bodies release endorphins and other stress-reducing hormones. As stress is released, we can feel our whole being lift…body, mind, and spirit.

Many people end the day with prayer, silence, or with inspirational reading. Very good ideas. Along with that you may want to keep at your bedside, for a last-of-the-day spirit lift:

- **a book of clean jokes**

- **a book of humorous stories or essays**

You will feel the last of the day's stresses ease away…and fall asleep with a more peaceful spirit.

3. Book of Proverbs 17:22 NKJV

5

The Diet Cure

"We had oriental food at the office party, and about an hour later my head hurt so bad I actually got dizzy and became violently ill. It was a nightmare. Someone told me it was probably the MSG they put in that stuff."

"I like to drink wine with meals. But I know I can't. The sulfites they add kill me. Even a few sips, and pretty soon my head is pounding."

Many of us are aware that certain food additives can trigger headaches and migraines. We've heard all the warnings about reducing salt intake, so that sodium intake won't wreak havoc with our blood pressure. Maybe you're also aware that the additive monosodium glutamate (MSG), which flavors many foods, can also trigger killer headaches.

But most of us are unaware that a whole range of foods, themselves, can trigger headaches. Moreover, for certain people, eating *itself* can be a source of headache pain.

Eating and Headaches

Medical researchers have discovered that there is a physical condition involving the intestines that can be a hidden trigger of headache and migraine suffering. In particular, they've found a link between intestinal damage and headaches. Here's how it works.

Overgrowths of certain yeasts, fungi, protozoa, or bacteria can cause an erosion in the intestinal lining. These include common fungi such as *Candida albicans* (which resembles a yeast), and outside invaders, such as the protozoan *Giardia lambia* (usually from drinking contaminated water). Certain medical conditions also cause erosion of the intestinal lining—including food poisoning, diverticulitis, celiac disease, Crohn's disease, and autoimmune disorders such as rheumatoid arthritis and lupus. Under these conditions the intestinal wall occasionally becomes raw, and minute perforations open up.

When food is introduced from the stomach into the intestines it is still only partway through the digestive cycle. When this partially digested food enters into a section of the intestines that is distressed and in a period of flare-up, it's possible for tiny food particles and acids from the digestive process to enter the bloodstream through those tiny perforations. These rogue food particles can cause the blood vessels to react and constrict, resulting in an excruciating headache.

Now that you're aware that a connection between intestinal distress and headaches can exist, you may want to watch for the onset of a headache or migraine after you eat. This would occur, of course, several hours after a meal rather than immediately after.

To treat overgrowths, and in cases of recurring intestinal distress—especially when bleeding is detected—you should seek a doctor's help.

Food Allergies

Food allergies provide more potential triggers for headaches and migraines.

In many cases, food allergies are quick and relatively easy to detect. You eat a meal, and within as little as 15 minutes you may experience a reaction. In these cases, the body's histamines and antibodies have been sent out into the blood on high alert. Reactions are obvious, usually coming in the form of *hives, rashes, swellings, vomiting, increased heart-rate, reddening of the skin (flushing), and sudden tiredness or weakness.*

Food allergies that result in headaches or migraines are a bit harder to detect. That's because about 70 percent of the body's immune system is located in the lower digestive tract—that is, in the small and large intestines. It takes several hours for food to clear the stomach and reach this area, and so our reaction time to any food that triggers a headache naturally takes longer.

In this same vein, perhaps the biggest reason certain food allergies are hard to detect is that over time, our awareness has moved away from food to other matters. In the space of a couple hours a lot can change. We may change locations, and if we start to feel bad two hours after a meal we're more likely to associate it with something in our immediate surroundings. ("Maybe the smell of her cologne is giving me a headache.") We become involved in other activities. ("Gosh, a little bit of digging in the garden and my head is splitting.") Maybe enough time has passed that we're now munching on a snack. ("Wow, that salty popcorn must have made my blood pressure jump, because my head is pounding.")

The point is, a couple of hours into a busy morning and breakfast can seem like ancient history. Jam an afternoon with a full agenda, and you might not even be able to remember what you had for lunch.

For this reason, if you're trying to track a headache, it's a good idea for you to keep close watch on your food intake.

Strategy #1 : Use a Food Journal

Using a Food Journal to detect headache triggers is a very simple matter. Whether you're trying to detect the presence of a food allergy for your own reasons or because you intend to seek help from a physician, having a daily record of what and when you eat is essential.

You will need:

- a spiral or loose-leaf notebook

- a commitment to recording everything you eat for a minimum of two weeks.

To help you set up your notebook pages, take a look at this sample entry:

Food Journal

Date: X/ Y/ ZZ

Breakfast: coffee w/cream & artificial sweetener; a bagel w/plain cream cheese

A.M. Snack: 2 cups of coffee w/cream and artificial sweetener

Lunch: deli sandwich w/roast beef and cheese; small bag of chips; 1 can diet cola

P.M. Snack: 1 can diet cola

Dinner: pasta w/tomato sauce, sausage, and parmesan; small green salad w/vinaigrette; ice water; sherbet

Evening Snack: fruit juice

Reactions: As usual, felt a headache coming on as I drove to work. Headachy all day until after dinner. The headache left, but I felt wiped out and cranky from all-day headache.

Notice how brief the entries can be, while still giving thorough information.

Incidentally, this headache sufferer has given some big clues as to what may be triggering his pain. His first dietary move would be to try eliminating caffeinated drinks and/or artificial sweeteners, since his headache appears to have gone away when he stopped consuming them and switched to drinking water and fruit juice.

Anytime we increase awareness of ourselves, our habits, and our reactions to our environment, we're taking an important step toward well-being. Why? Because personal awareness is always the first step toward making healthy changes.

Strategy #2: Find and Eliminate Problem Foods

If foods are triggering your headaches and migraines you will need to try a simple elimination diet. Here's how it works:

Step One: For two weeks, compile lists.

- Make a list of the foods you eat in a two-week period. This isn't as difficult as it sounds because most of us "graze" within a surprisingly small range and eat only about 10 or 12 different foods.

- Make a separate list of additives in the prepared foods you eat, including all additives such as preservatives, cooking oils, vitamins, minerals, and herbs.
- Make a third list of any and all supplements you're taking.

Step Two: Choose one of the foods you eat most often and eliminate it from your diet for one week. Carefully note in your Food Journal the date you start your elimination. Also note any reactions you notice.

In particular, you are watching for headache-free patterns to emerge.

Step Three: At the end of a week, if there's no change in your headache patterns, you may want to add that particular food back into your diet. Then you'll choose another of your most-eaten foods to eliminate for the coming week.

Although this is a simple strategy, it can take time. You do want to be thorough and observant.

To help you zero-in a little more quickly, though, what follows is a list of foods known to cause food allergies and/or trigger headaches and migraines.

One at a time, try eliminating these.

Foods That Can Trigger Headaches

- *Alcohol.* Alcohol causes rapid changes in your blood vessels, and it affects the central nervous system. These variations can cause terrible headaches.

- *Avocados.* Although nutritionists find many reasons to consider avocados to be a "perfect food," they contain *tyrosine*, a nitrogen compound that can trigger headaches.

- *Chocolate.* This beloved treat sadly contains a substance called *phenylethylamine*, another nitrogen compound known to be a source of headache pain.

- *Coffee and Colas (and "the Caffeine Contradiction").* The caffeine in coffee and cola drinks can affect some of us as powerfully as a drug. Not only is it a stimulant, it acts as a vascular dilator, meaning that it causes your veins to expand. This can trigger a headache for some people...and ease a headache for others.

- *Beer.* Beer contains *tyramine*...a third kind of nitrogen compound. This one can irritate blood vessels in the brain and trigger excruciating migraines.

- *Citrus Fruits.* Oranges, limes, grapefruits, lemons—fruits in this family contain nitrogen compounds of a kind that can trigger pain by constricting blood vessels throughout the cardiovascular system.

- *Cured Meats.* Bacon, bologna, cured hams, hotdogs, sausages—all these are loaded with sodium nitrite...which produces killer headaches in some people. But in fact, other processed meats can also contain sodium nitrite. *If you suspect this additive is a problem for you, read the labels on all packaged and processed meats.*

- *Milk and milk products.* A substantial number of people cannot tolerate the lactose in milk and other milk-based products. Most experience nausea and other digestive problems. Studies also show that a portion of lactose-intolerant people also experience severe headaches, making this one of those foods you may want to eliminate first to see what happens. Just be aware that lactose can be found in numerous food items.

- *Monosodium Glutamate (MSG).* Although this substance is popularly associated with Chinese food, it's also used to promote freshness in salad bars and in some fast foods, including chicken and burgers. If you eat out and you know or suspect that MSG is a headache trigger, ask your waiter if they use it in their food preparations. Unfortunately, now that MSG is getting something of a bad rap, it can be disguised on labels as "hydrolyzed protein" or the catchall... "natural flavorings."

- *Legumes and Nuts.* If you are heavy on bean, pea, and nut intake for some reason, you may have to make some serious rearrangements in your diet. These foods contain nitrogen compounds, a known cause of headaches and migraines.

  Nuts are often a greater problem than beans or peas for headache sufferers. First, nuts are naturally rich in their own oils and therefore contain more nitrogen than other legumes. Second, they're usually eaten roasted, not boiled, so nitrogens aren't lost to the "pot liquor."

- *Onions.* Contain nitrogen compounds.

- *Pickled Foods.* Anything pickled—from cucumbers, to eggs, to herrings—can be a potential trigger.

- *Wines.* As noted at the opening of this chapter, most wines contain sulfites, though you can purchase some that do not. Red wines, in particular, contain *tyramine,* so those affected by wine are getting a double whammy of sulfites and nitrogen compounds.

- *Ripened Cheeses.* Let's start with the *safe* cheeses. The milder white ones—such as American, baby Swiss, Havarti, Gouda, farmer's cheese, mozzarella…also cream cheese and cottage cheese—these are unlikely to be a problem.

  The cheeses that are likely to cause trouble are the aged or "ripened" ones. These include all varieties of blue cheese, Brie, Camembert, the cheddars, and Gruyére.

- *Sauerkraut.* If you like Reuben sandwiches and 'kraut on your hotdogs, you may be out of luck. Like other foods produced by fermentation, sauerkraut is a possible trigger food. Kimchee—that fermented cabbage "delight" omnipresent in Asian restaurants—is definitely off-limits.

- *Sour Cream.* Fermentation makes this dairy product (also **buttermilk**) a problem for many headache and migraine sufferers.

- *Sugar Substitutes.* In particular, we're talking **aspartame.** As you know, this artificial sweetener is found in diet soft drinks. But it's also creeping into other food substances.

Rx

READ LABELS, READ LABELS...
READ LABELS

∼

Processed foods prove the truth of the old saying, "The devil is in the details."

Some of us have trained ourselves to look for the obvious on food labels—such as the amount of fat, protein, or carbohydrates...or the cholesterol content. Maybe we should dig a little deeper and check out all the ingredients if we're concerned about the presence of potential headache triggers. Many seemingly innocent processed foods harbor "hidden" ingredients that can create health problems.

Be sure you read all "nutrition facts" and all the ingredients. Here's what you might find:

- A can of "healthy" chunky soup contains **39 percent** of the FDA's recommended daily allotment of **sodium**. What does that much sodium do, hitting your cardiovascular system all at once? Then there's the second wallop, from **MSG**.

- A can of cut green beans, and another can of butter beans...a healthy choice, right?—Both contain **MSG**.

- Little pasta shapes with meatballs, in a can. The label announces: "Good source of protein!" With an unbelievable **41 percent** of the RDA of **sodium**...and with "natural flavors" that likely include MSG...this is potentially a good source for a bad headache.

- A box of flavored rice...a box of instant potatoes....Buried down there in the dozens of substances (whatever happened to just a little butter?) is a load of both **MSG** and **sulfites**. If you want a highly nutritious, starchy carb to go with dinner, try Quaker Pearled Barley, which contains (are you ready?) just pearled barley—one of the best plant-based, protein-carb mixes you can eat.

Do you *really* know what you're eating? *Read those labels.*

- *Tea.* Caffeine, of course, is the problem. Trade off for the low-caffeine and herbal teas, and you'll be fine.

Finally...

- *Foods with tiny seeds.* As we've seen, rawness in the intestinal tract can result in headaches. For this reason, you may wish to stop eating strawberries, raspberries, kiwi fruit and other fruits or berries...also foods made with sesame seeds...to see if these eliminations have a beneficial effect.

Okay, so if you eliminate many of these foods from your diet, you're giving up almost everything that makes life worth living— right? Not to fear. It's highly unlikely you'll have to eliminate all of these foods, only some of them. On the "big-plus side," an elimination diet can help you target headache triggers that you might otherwise overlook for a long time.

If some foods trigger headaches—are there foods that can actually help prevent them? The answer is...*yes.*

Strategy #3: Add Headache-Preventing Foods

Many of our headaches and migraines are triggered by rapid changes in our cardiovascular system. We can suffer when blood vessels rapidly dilate or constrict, either one.

For this reason, many headache and migraine sufferers find it very helpful to eat diets rich in foods that help keep the cardiovascular system stable.

These include:

- **Foods Rich in Vitamin A:** This vitamin is an important antioxidant, and its ability to enhance cardiovascular health makes it very important in the diet of headache sufferers. You will want to eat fruits with red, yellow, and orange meats, such as:

cantaloupes	*peaches*
mangoes	*plums*
oranges	*watermelon*
papaya	

Also red, yellow, and orange vegetables, including:

beets	*pumpkin*
bell peppers	*squash*
carrots	*waxed beans*

- *Foods Rich in the B Vitamins.* The more stress we experience, the more our need increases for the whole family of B vitamins. When we're low on B vitamins our muscles tense and lose flexibility. They tend to tighten and clench the nerves that radiate through them. When this occurs—especially in the shoulders, upper back, neck, and face—the result is a dull, headachy feeling...or a full-blown muscle-tension headache.

Foods you'll want to eat to pump in the B vitamins include:

broccoli	*barley*	*brussels sprouts*
millet	*brown rice*	*rye*
chard	*liver*	*kale*
kidney	*spinach*	*eggs*
cabbage	*parsley*	

- *Foods Rich in Vitamin C.* Very important for cardiovascular health. Most fruits are rich in vitamin C, especially berries. But you will want to be careful with berries that have those tiny seeds that can irritate the intestinal lining.

- *Foods Rich in Selenium.* This trace mineral, important to circulatory health, was once in rich supply in most of our foods. But because overfarming has stripped soils of their natural traces, many of us who think we're eating a pretty good, or even excellent, diet are often low in selenium intake.

Selenium rich foods include:

fish	*garlic*
liver	*sesame oil*

- *Foods Rich in Zinc.* Zinc is another trace mineral that is often depleted in headache sufferers. Like selenium, we require only tiny amounts—not even milligrams but *micrograms*—of zinc. But stress—and a diet consisting of processed foods—will rapidly deplete our bodies of this mineral.

Among the most common zinc-rich foods are:

almonds	*buckwheat*
shellfish	*rye*
spelt	

THE INCREDIBLE APPLE

～

Despite the whole Garden of Eden thing, the apple is one of God's great gifts to us.

Apples can be important in the diet of headache sufferers whose triggers have to do with intestinal and digestive problems and toxins in the bloodstream.

How so?

- **Apples encourage the growth of beneficial bacteria in the large intestine. These bacteria combat unhealthy overgrowths of harmful bacteria, which restores balance to our system and allows raw or inflamed tissue to heal.**

- **A substance in apples (pectin) helps to remove toxic metals and other chemicals in the bloodstream.**

As an important side benefit, apple pectin can also reduce serum cholesterol levels significantly.

- *Yogurt.* Real yogurt—the kind made with active cultures—helps restore the balance of good bacteria in the intestines. Good bacteria, the kind we need for healthy digestion, are not only wiped out by incursions of bad bacteria...they are also devastated by stress, smoking, alcohol, antacid use, and, of course, antibiotics. Eating yogurt helps reduce overall stress on the body...and also reduces the risk of vascular headaches.

Just in Case

As you can see, attention to diet is very important for many physiological reasons. Changes in diet to avoid "trigger" foods and add preventative ones can make a huge difference for headache and migraine sufferers. Paying attention to what, and how, we eat is also an important way to develop a new kind of self-awareness...and that in itself is important if we want to experience good health and overall well-being.

We all know, however, that it's not always possible to eat a healthy diet consistently. Our schedules get crazy. We're out on the road, starving, with nothing healthy to eat in sight. Besides that, some of the beneficial foods listed above may not agree with you...or you may just plain not like them.

For those situations in which you can't get the health benefits you need from a good diet, you may want to consider using natural supplements. Some in particular provide help for headache and migraine sufferers. You'll find the latest information on headache-relieving supplements in the next chapter.

6

Natural Supplements

Some of the supplements discussed in this chapter may react with certain medications. Others may have adverse effects on various health conditions such as pregnancy, high blood pressure, depressive disorders, and others. As yet we do not have full knowledge of which herbs may react negatively when taken with other herbs.

Some, but not all, contraindications are mentioned.

When you are taking supplements, you are wise to consult your healthcare professional to create a health plan that is safe and right for you.

*I*n the not-too-distant past, natural supplements were considered to be on the "fringe" of healthcare. You bought them in funky little stores from a man or woman who was drinking hot goat's milk and wearing a tie-dyed tee shirt.

These days, supplements are often referred to as "natural medicines." And they're everywhere—in our grocery stores, pharmacies, discount chains. They're even creeping into our foods, as the labels on soft drinks and "healthy snacks" proudly proclaim: "With Ginseng!" or "Contains St. John's Wort!"

As natural supplements have come into popular usage, of course, many big claims are being made—among them, that certain substances can cure, or at least greatly reduce, headache and migraine suffering.

The Skeptics

Some skeptics may not consider natural supplements as a viable way to treat health needs. Some doctors and other healthcare professionals are dubious about them, too.

For one thing, they say, not enough studies have been done on either the effectiveness of most supplements or on their long-term effects. Besides that, quality control can vary greatly from product to product—or even between one lot and another from the same manufacturer. Some studies have shown that any given capsule of supplement may contain *more* than the dosage stated on the label...or *much less*...or even *none at all*.

If that's the case, how can you regulate doses in a way that offers any therapeutic benefit?

Response

In response to the demands of consumers and healthcare professionals, manufacturers of natural supplements have learned to pay more careful attention to the quality and consistency of their products. Some have their own laboratories, while others use independent labs, to test products for potency, consistency, and purity.

Some supplement manufacturers also make information available to consumers about possible negative reactions to their product. For this reason, reading labels has become more important than in the past. Beyond that, websites now exist where consumers can look up information about supplement manufacturers and how their products rate. For product ratings, a good source to consult is: **www.consumerlab.com.**

Mostly, though, in response to skeptics, the people who produce natural supplements *and* those who use them make their stand on this ground: *Natural supplements work.*

Admittedly, they say, the proof for the effectiveness of supplements is largely based on "anecdotal evidence"—that is, the word of people who claim to have been cured, or experienced improvement, by using a particular supplement to treat a health problem. That's good enough, many say, to warrant giving herbs, minerals, and vitamins a try. Furthermore, the growing crowd of supplement users say that natural medicines can work *just as effectively* as synthetic pharmaceuticals *without* the damaging side effects that occur with many drugs.

In fact there *is* growing medical evidence to support the claims that natural medicines work. What these researchers are doing, in many cases, is actually *re*discovering the effectiveness of natural remedies our culture forgot about. Often, the only reason we stopped using, for instance, healing herbs is that someone found a way to produce synthetically, in a laboratory, the naturally occurring chemical compounds that make the herbs effective.

Here, then, is a selection of herbs, minerals, vitamins, and other natural medicines you may wish to try. If you approach the process carefully and pay attention, you will learn which treatments can work as headache and migraine remedies for you.

A Small Apothecary
of Headache and Migraine Remedies
ᖰᖰᖰ

The Ayurvedic Shelf

Many doctors trained in traditional western (allopathic) medicine, as well as complementary health practitioners, are beginning to use traditional Indian techniques in the treatment of some ailments, including headaches and migraines. These techniques are part of a centuries-old set of practices collectively known as Ayurvedic medicine.

Though even the word "Ayurvedic" sounds exotic to western ears, the substances used are natural, derived from plant and mineral sources. Many who have relied on powerful headache-relief medicines find they are amazed at how effective these simple remedies can be. When selecting a treatment, you must give consideration to the type of headache you are experiencing.

- **"Dry Headache"**—that is, a dull headache accompanied by thirst and tiredness or exhaustion. The cause of "dry headaches" may be dehydration, as elevation of electrolytes relieves the pain.

Treatment: Sip one pint of water mixed with ¼ teaspoon sea salts, one tablespoon of sugar, and the juice of half a lime. Repeat every 45 to 60 minutes until the headache subsides.

- **"Shooting, Piercing Headache"**—during which the pain is felt behind the eyes, stabbing deep into the head, often accompanied by nausea that can range from light to heavy. These headaches are often connected to stomach and intestinal problems.

Treatment: Dissolve sandalwood powder (available at Indian groceries and some healthfood stores) with a little water to make a paste. Apply to your forehead and temples and allow it to dry completely before rinsing off. This poultice will help ease tension in the small muscles of the face. If your stomach will tolerate it, eat something mild and/or lightly sweetened—for instance, crackers or rice pudding. The crackers will help absorb excess stomach acids, as will the rice, while being easy to digest. A small amount of sugar will alleviate "sour stomach."

- **"Headaches that occur seasonally, or at a certain time of day, and get worse when you bend over."** These are probably associated with allergies, or with sinus congestion. Sometimes people who suffer with "sinus headaches" find that neither prescription nor over-the-counter medications help. Ayurvedic practitioners suggest you try the following combination of remedies.

Treatment: Pour one cup of boiling water into a large mug. Make a tea of one pinch of ground cloves, ½ teaspoon of ground ginger, and one teaspoon of ground cinnamon. This combination of spices has a number of stimulating properties. The aromatic effects help to open the sinuses, encouraging drainage. The compounds within these spices, when they enter the bloodstream, increase circulation by dilating blood vessels, fight infection, and also stimulate the sinuses to open and drain.

Also:

Make a saline mixture in these proportions: $\frac{1}{8}$ teaspoon of sea salt to one tablespoon of warm water. Using a dropper, inject the solution into each nostril a drop or two at a time. A warm, mild, saline solution will continue the work of healing within the sinus cavities.

The Herb Shelf

Herbs offer a gentle way to counter the imbalances within our bodies that can trigger pain. Because most herbs work in a gentle way, the temptation is to think they aren't strong enough or don't work fast enough to ease headaches and migraines. We are indeed a "quick relief" culture—even if that relief is costly to us in many ways.

Those who try herbal remedies, however, soon discover that they can be as effective as pharmaceutical painkillers while avoiding the side effects.

Three important secrets to success in using herbal remedies are:

1. **Develop that all-important awareness of yourself and the things that are likely to trigger your headaches.**

When you know that a triggering situation is unavoidable, you can then use healing herbs in advance as a preventative.

2. **Develop a habit of using pain-relieving herbs as teas and in foods.**

By using herbs more frequently you can maintain a sort of "baseline level" of their active, pain-relieving ingredients in your system. When you feel a headache or migraine coming on, a "booster" dose will help you reach the therapeutic level more quickly.

3. **Give herbs time to work.**

It can take 10 to 20 days for the active agents in most herbs to reach a therapeutic level in your body. Some herbs will have more immediate effects, of course, and you can use them on the spot when you feel a headache coming on. Still, they are more effective when used regularly, and their active ingredients are present for a longer time in your body.

Here are some individual herbs, and also some herbal tea remedies, known to prevent or relieve headache pain. Some are available in both dry form and in tinctures.

- *Feverfew.* This herb was considered something of a "wonder drug" back in the days when people understood the medicinal properties of herbs. In the 1772 edition of his *Family Herbal,* John Hill, a renowned expert in natural medicines, states, "[For curing] the worst headache, this herb exceeds every other treatment that is known." Well before him, the great sixteenth-century herbalist, Gerard, wrote that besides curing headaches feverfew was highly recommended "for them that are...melancholic, sad, or pensive."

  Modern studies have supported Hill's and Gerard's assertions. Regular use of feverfew decreases the level of prostaglandins in the blood. Though these hormones are naturally occurring in the body, overproduction seems to trigger cramps and severe headaches. Because feverfew reduces prostaglandin levels, this accounts for its pain-relieving property.

  Additionally, feverfew has calming properties, making it a good choice when we are in an agitated state. It is widely used, therefore, in cases of stress- or anxiety-induced depression. This herb is available in capsules and in a tincture.

  Warning: Feverfew acts as a blood thinner, so you should avoid this if you are on any blood-thinning medication such as Coumadin®, Warfarin, Heparin, and some pain killers...including the regular use of common aspirin.

- *Ginger.* Ginger also works by reducing prostaglandins, but seems to be gentler than other herbs. This makes it a good choice for those who suffer more from those dull, chronic, muscle-tension headaches.

  Those who use ginger on a daily basis find that it is a powerful preventative. This spice is one of the easiest to add to your regular diet because of its delightful flavor. Raw gingerroot is, of course, stronger and can be used like its powdered counterpart to make healing teas and in cooking.

If you don't favor the taste of ginger—or just don't want to taste it all that often—ginger is available in capsule form. You can also carry it with you in its crystalized form and eat it when you feel a headache coming on. Some have reported feeling its positive effects in only 30 minutes.

- *Gingko.* First studies on the use of gingko in headache relief have been impressive. It has a more marked effect than ginger. Some 80 percent of those suffering migraines and cluster headaches report marked improvement. Gingko can also be used to treat tinnitus (ringing in the ears) and dizziness (due to vertigo).

  Like feverfew, gingko is considered by many practitioners of natural medicine to be an "herb of choice" in treating headaches and migraines. Although it reduces prostaglandin levels and relaxes vascular tension it does not act as a blood thinner, making it a better choice for some.

  Gingko is available in capsules and in a tincture.

- *Meadowsweet.* The word "aspirin" comes from spirea, which is an alternate name for meadowsweet. What's the connection? Meadowsweet contains salicin, which the body converts to salicylic acid, which is the active ingredient in aspirin.

  Here's the thing about aspirin. It was introduced by the Bayer Company in the late 1800s...before government regulatory agencies existed. The aspirin we take these days is such a strong drug—because today's version delivers a synthetic form of salicylic acid directly into the stomach—that in the opinion of many medical researchers, if it were just being discovered today, it would have to be regulated and made available only by prescription. But it's not, and so its damaging effects can be too easily overlooked. Because it's purchased over the counter, we consumers don't recognize how strong its effects on the body really are.

Coming back to meadowsweet....This herb gives us a much gentler, safer alternative to aspirin. It offers the body salicin, and allows the body to convert this natural substance slowly, naturally, into the pain reliever, salicylic acid. Yes, it may take a few minutes longer for the herb to counter your headache, but it's also less destructive to your stomach lining and less of a shock to your system because its healing agents enter the bloodstream more gradually.

Meadowsweet tea is a common way to ingest this herb, which is available in dried form and in a tincture.

- *Skullcap.* The effectiveness of this herb—also known as Chinese skullcap—as a pain reliever has been compared to the powerful drug phenylbutazone—but it doesn't create the damage that long-term uses of the drug causes.

Skullcap works by reducing inflammation of the sheath that lines and otherwise protects the nerves. As an anti-inflammatory it is every bit as effective as aspirin or ibuprofen and doesn't upset or irritate the stomach as these substances often do.

Skullcap can be taken in capsule form or in a tincture.

- *Vervain.* When your headaches are due to overworked, stressed, or strained muscles, vervain may be your treatment of choice. When muscles are stressed, the result is constricted or "pinched" nerves. Vervain works by encouraging the regeneration of muscle tissue and nerve cells.

If you have experienced injuries to the nerves in the shoulders, upper back, or neck—even old injuries—you can benefit from the regenerative effects of this herb.

Vervain comes in both capsule and tincture form.

- *Willowbark* is another powerful, natural inflammatory. Its active ingredient is salicin, and so it acts to relieve headache and migraine pain much the same as meadowsweet, reducing prostaglandin in the blood.

TWO HERBAL HEADACHE "ELIXIRS"

∾

Remedy #1:

One of the most effective remedies for a headache or migraine is made of herbal tinctures, which can be mixed in advance and kept on hand for use when you first detect the onset of pain. Many keep the following mixture in small brown bottles—the kind that come with a dropper in the screw-on cap—and store it in their cupboard or medicine chest. You can also carry it in your purse or briefcase.

To make this remedy, mix one teaspoon each of these tinctures:

feverfew	*peppermint*	*ginger*
ginkgo	*valerian*	

Before or during a headache, take a dropperful on the tongue, as needed. Up to eight times a day.

Remedy #2:

This is a remedy that can become part of your daily regimen, which makes it a good "preventative" medicine. The addition of mint makes it a flavorful, refreshing drink, too.

In a jar or canister mix a tea blend from one part each of these dried herbs:

wintergreen

willowbark

meadowsweet

Place one teaspoon of this blend in a tea ball. Pour boiling water over it in a cup, and let it steep for six to seven minutes…or as much as ten minutes if you like a stronger cup of tea.

The Mineral Shelf

When illness or overwork stresses the body, we can become deficient in important minerals that keep the muscle and circulatory functions healthy. Mineral deficiency can result in numerous physical problems, of course—and one is that it can trigger excruciating headaches.

A blood screen can tell you if you are mineral deficient, and which minerals to increase. Hair analysis, though sometimes discounted by allopathic medical practitioners, can also give you a reading.

In general, people whose headaches or migraines are triggered by mineral deficiencies most often benefit by increasing their intake of the following minerals.

- *Calcium-Magnesium.* It is important to take these two minerals in combination, as each helps with the absorption and use of the other. For this reason, they are often sold in combination, which takes the guesswork out of how much of each you should take. The chelated form of these minerals is the best.

- *Potassium.* You will want to take no more than 90 to 100 mg a day. The reason is, potassium and sodium need to be kept in balance in the body. The average diet tends to give us more than enough sodium. We tend to get less potassium in our diets, and potassium can easily be drained from our system when we experience physical or emotional stress. The bottom line is, when this balance is thrown off our muscles lose flexibility and tighten, putting pressure on the nerves…also resulting in that "stressed out" feeling doctors refer to as "hypertension"—an intense feeling of stress and pressure that won't let up.

To restore the sodium-potassium balance we need to supplement with only a relatively small amount of potassium.

HOMEOPATHY

∿

Decades ago, homeopathic remedies were widely used in the United States and Europe. In the States their popularity went into a rapid decline when synthetic drugs came on the scene, and for a time they were consigned to the realm of "quackery." In Europe, however, homeopathy continued to develop. Now, as this alternative therapy makes a comeback on the west side of the Atlantic, homeopathic medicines and their use have been refined by years of modern European research and trials.

Homeopathic medicines are now widely available and often come in the form of powders. Many homeopathic doctors insist, however, that the right substances and doses must be used in order for the treatment to be effective. A practitioner will be able to adjust the doses, they claim, by carefully observing how they affect you.

Substances used in treating headaches and migraines include:

Aconite	Glonoine	Iris
Apis	Ignatia	Sanguinaria
Belladonna		

The Vitamin Shelf

Vitamin deficiencies are commonly known to cause a variety of maladies and conditions from skin problems to bad circulation…from fatigue to depression…from brittle nails to hair loss. It's less commonly known that vitamin deficiencies can also trigger headaches and migraines.

As is true with minerals, vitamin deficiencies can result from stress or illness. The deficiency creates conditions in our muscle and vascular systems that can trigger the pain that lays us low.

There's an additional problem, though. When we become deficient, just consuming a normal amount of vitamins is often not enough to replenish our body's lowered supplies. In other words, for a time we will need to take *more* of the vitamin we're missing to get us caught up. And if we experience long-term stress or illness, we will need more vitamins *all* the time to keep our resources at the proper level.

Here are the vitamins often used in the practice of natural medicine to prevent or relieve headache pain.

- *Vitamin A (Beta-carotene).* Many headaches and migraines are triggered by vision problems, including common problems like poor eyesight, and also the more serious ones like macular degeneration or glaucoma. We can also suffer when eyestrain from overwork, poor lighting, or too bright lighting puts a strain on the ocular nerves. Vitamin A is nature's "tonic" for the eyes.

  Vitamin A is also a powerful antioxidant, which means that it "scours" the blood of free radicals. Its help in maintaining our vascular health makes it an ally in headache prevention.

  Although vitamin A in higher doses has proven to be helpful to some headache and migraine sufferers, you should be careful to flush your system with water if you are taking this vitamin. Though you would have to take quite a bit, over a long period of time for vitamin-A toxicity to occur, it's better to be safe than sorry.

- *Vitamin C.* The esterized form of this important vitamin (sold as Ester-C) is the type you want. Vitamin C is essential in so many of the body's functions—from synthesizing food, to strengthening immunity, to tissue and cell repair, to cleansing the blood of free radicals and other invaders—it would be hard to list the many ways this powerful substance is useful as a deterrent to headache and migraine suffering.

  Like the rest of the vitamins that follow in this list, vitamin C is water soluble, which means the body does not store it in its fat cells. In other words, it doesn't stick around long and therefore needs to be replenished frequently…even daily. It also means it can be taken in relatively high doses each day without causing problems. Dr. Linus Pauling, who championed the cause of vitamin C as a natural medicine, took up to 100,000 mg of it a day!

Many who take vitamin C for therapeutic reasons, not just as a "daily booster," take between 3,000 and 10,000 mg a day—far short of Dr. Pauling's record, but very effective nonetheless.

- *Vitamin E* is one of the most important vitamins necessary for maintaining a healthy cardiovascular system. It helps clean the blood of free radicals, just like A and C, the other antioxidants. Beyond that, it also aids in the repair of cell walls and the creation of new cells, which means it helps keep blood vessels supple and nerves in fine working order.

All these facts make vitamin E important in the prevention of several conditions that trigger headaches and migraines.

- *Vitamin B$_2$ (Riboflavin).* Stress rapidly depletes all the B vitamins from the body. The result is muscle tension and nerve inflammation. Increasing the intake of B$_2$ has been shown to decrease the need for anti-inflammatories and to effectively relieve headache pain.

- *Vitamin B$_3$ (Niacin, Niacinamide).* When the eyes are overworked and strained, they can become extremely photosensitive, further irritating the optic nerve. B$_3$ can be highly effective in treating headaches produced by eyestrain.

- *Vitamin B$_6$ (Pyridoxine).* B$_6$ may be helpful in relieving headaches that are triggered by various causes.

This vitamin aids in the digestion of food, particularly proteins. This makes it a useful supplement for those whose headaches are related to digestive or intestinal problems. It can counter the effects of some food additives, for instance the MSG that is fairly omnipresent in processed foods.

B$_6$ is also helpful in regulating the production of many hormones, which makes it a valuable ally for women who experience headaches and severe cramping during their menstrual cycle.

If you are photosensitive because of eyestrain, or your nervous system has been stressed for any other reason, B_6 is a wonderful "tonic" and restorative for the nerve cells.

℞

AROMATHERAPY

∼

Just mention "aromatherapy" and many people in the traditional medical community will roll their eyes. Nonetheless, a wide range of aromas have a reputation for relieving headache pain.

At least part of the reason aromatherapy is successful may be that it encourages deep breathing. That, of course, oxygenates the blood and increases circulation. The more we center-in on our breathing, too, the more likely we are to trigger the body's "deep relaxation" response. This releases many of the body's own health-promoting chemicals, such as endorphins…all of which relax muscle tension. Besides all that, you could do worse things when you have a headache than to lie down in a soft-lit room, breathe deeply, and take a break.

The scents listed below are often used specifically to help relieve the pain of even the most terrible headaches.

Betony   Peppermint   Melissa

Lavender   Wintergreen

To enjoy their benefits, you can mix drops of these oils with your bathwater. Or you can mix them with water in a spray bottle and mist a room. You can also place a few drops into a small, clay apparatus that rests on a common lightbulb. (These are usually available where aroma oils are sold.) As the clay warms up, the scent is diffused into the air.

An important caution:

Although aromatherapy seems innocent enough, its effects can be powerful—so strong, in fact, that certain scents have been known to induce labor. In people with certain health conditions, they may cause other physiological reactions.

For this reason, it's best to consult with someone experienced in aromatherapy before using the oils.

Those Are the Natural Medicines,
These Are the Guidelines

If you are going to use the natural medicines listed above for their therapeutic benefit, it's important that you treat them *as* medicines. A casual attitude won't help you, and in certain cases it could cause you problems.

A few simple but important guidelines apply:

1. If you are taking a prescription medication, check with your physician and/or pharmacist to see if your medication is known to react negatively with the supplement(s) you're planning to try.

2. Keep track of the supplements you take, including the date on which you started and your daily dosage. You can simply write this on a piece of paper and keep it in your medicine cabinet. Or if you keep a journal, such as the Food Journal recommended in the previous chapter, record the information there. Why is this important?

- If your headaches subside you'll want a record of exactly what you were taking, and when, and how much.

- If you experience a serious illness, a medical emergency, or require surgery, your healthcare practitioners will need to know exactly what you have been taking and the dosages. Remember, any supplement can have a potentially negative reaction with a pharmaceutical drug.

3. Get in the habit of drinking water to flush your system. When you are taking medications—even natural ones—keep the water flowing to help cleanse the liver and kidneys.

4. If you experience a reaction, *stop taking the supplement immediately*. Flush your system with water. Call your physician or pharmacist to determine if there are other steps you should take to safeguard your well-being.

5. Give it time. Natural medicines *do* work—often not as quickly as pharmaceuticals. But as many are discovering, they work just as effectively.

7

Body Basics

*F*or many people, headaches and migraines are triggered by structural problems in their physical bodies. These problems, which affect body mechanics, can include:

- muscle strains and muscle spasms

- misalignment of bones

- stressed nerves

- stressed blood vessels

The result is that stress in the body affects the nerves, muscles, and blood vessels in the neck and head...often causing one terrible headache after another, unless the stress point is found and the stress is released.

Avoidance Is the Wrong Solution

Most people who suffer body-stress headaches and migraines notice that engaging in heavy work, exercise, and play, or even sexual activity can trigger their pain. Our tendency, then, is to avoid these things, only to find that heavy work is sometimes unavoidable... and life without good exercise and play equals weight gain, lousy moods, frequent depressions, and sluggish digestion. And the inability to relax with a sexual partner robs us of the emotional intimacy we crave and works against a loving relationship.

We were created with physical bodies, and we need a whole variety of physical activities for overall well-being. Excusing our-selves from things like exercise, hard work, or sex is in fact the wrong plan. Because these activities, in themselves, contribute to good health we should assume that we *are* going to do them. What we need to figure out is *how* to stay active without triggering that head-splitting pain.

The problem for many headache and migraine sufferers is to find physical activity that will not itself trigger the pain. For some people, headaches can be caused by vigorous and especially jarring motions or by sudden stress placed on the cardiovascular system. For this reason, *slow and cautious* is a good rule of thumb when trying out a new physical regimen or pain-relief strategy. Light to moderate exercise is the best choice.

What follows are simple strategies we can use to ease the body stresses that result in headaches and migraines, beginning with the easiest and most basic.

Strategy #1: Better Breathing

Tony suffered from headaches that left him nauseous every time he lifted weights—even on days when he did a light workout. He thought the problem must be the result of a pinched nerve. When a trainer observed him, though, he spotted the real problem. "You're not breathing right at all. In fact, every time you [push the weights] you hold your breath. You're starving your body for oxygen and that's putting stress on your veins, your muscle tissues, your nerves…everything."

MaryBeth left work several days a week with a splitting headache. One day a co-worker passed her workstation and remarked, "How can you even breathe—sitting all hunched over like that?" When a naturopathic doctor taught her proper breathing techniques—and also what to do about muscle knots in her shoulders caused by poor posture—the headaches caused by those particular triggers stopped.

Poor breathing leaves us with sluggish circulation and poorly oxygenated blood. This has several very bad effects on the body. It puts stress on our vascular system, and it causes toxins to build up in our muscles, including acids that cause the muscles to spasm. We experience fatigue, tightness, and "muscle knots." When muscles tighten, the nerves passing through them can feel like they're being crushed in a vise.

Poorly oxygenated blood is responsible for another set of headache triggers, as well. When the blood is well oxygenated, the body is able to better produce and use hormones—that wide range of biochemicals that are so important to every bodily function. When our blood is low in oxygen, metabolism and the use of these vital substances is impaired. Women who suffer from headaches associated with their menstrual cycle, for instance, can benefit from learning the practice of proper breathing.

If you want to see what proper breathing looks like in a truly natural form, just watch an infant breathe: all tummy motion, with very little chest expansion. For some reason—possibly the onset of adult stresses, which cause us to "clench" in the middle and slow or hold our breath—we lose this very natural mode of breathing.

We can change the habit of poor breathing, however, with just a little conscious effort.

Do This:

1. *At least once a day, practice proper breathing. Begin by sitting comfortably, with your back straight, in a chair.* You can lean back a little in a semi-reclining position, if that will help you relax more. The thing is to keep your back straight.

2. *Breathe in slowly through your nose.* In an earlier chapter we tried a similar strategy to help establish a calmer mental or spiritual state. This time, keep your awareness focused on your body. In particular....

3. *Let your lungs fill...and your abdomen rise.* When you're breathing correctly, your diaphragm will expand more than your ribs, and you'll see your abdomen rise (like a baby's).

4. *Release the breath quickly through your mouth.* This allows the toxins to escape more rapidly from your body.

Notice the pattern: *In slowly* through your nose; *out quickly* through your mouth. The pattern itself will help you focus awareness on what you're doing, which will help you keep it going. The slow intake will not introduce oxygen into your blood too quickly, which would cause you to become light-headed. And the quick release helps trigger the deep relaxation response (so important to supporting overall immune function).

Keeping your blood oxygenated *and* your vascular system free from stress is a key to avoiding or relieving headaches. This strategy can also be helpful if eating has stressed your digestive tract and you are experiencing nausea or tension there.

Strategy #2: Stretch Away Tension

While we're going about our normal daily routines…and even while we're asleep…our muscles are gathering acids and other toxins produced by our body's biochemical processes. Even sitting at a desk, holding our head in roughly the same position all day, can leave our neck and upper shoulder muscles stiff.

As a result, our muscles become less flexible—just plain stiff, and "knotted." Here come the headaches.

Stretching is one of the simplest and most effective things you can do to release built-up tension from your body. Most of us engage in a five-second "yawn and stretch" from time to time…but not the total body stretch we really need to keep us limber. It's important to remember that any stretch exercise should end before you experience discomfort.

For stretches that will effectively release muscle tension before it builds to a headache or migraine…

Do This:

1. (Seated or standing.) Raise your arms straight above your head and clasp your hands. Then:

- Use your right hand to gently draw your left arm down and behind your head. Keep your left arm as straight as possible. Keep your back straight, too. Feel the muscles all around your left shoulder blade as they stretch and release tension. Hold…and release.

- Repeat for the benefit of the right side.

2. (Standing or seated.) With your left hand, reach across your chest and clasp the back side of your right elbow. Then:

- Gently pull your right arm up…and across your body to the left…until your upper right arm brushes the underside of your jaw. Hold until you feel the upper back muscles stretch…and then release.

- Repeat for your left side.

3. (Standing or seated.) Use your head. *Never roll your head in a circular motion, because it can cause severe and permanent damage to the small disks and vertebrae in your neck.* Instead:

- Lower your chin to your chest. In this position, gently move your chin from side to side like a pendulum…just far enough to feel the little muscles at the base of your skull stretch. Return your chin to your chest *before* raising your head.

- Now…gently lower your head to one side, as if to touch your ear to your shoulder. Return to upright and center.

- Repeat for the other side.

4. (Standing.) Loosen your back and legs. Gently, slowly bend from the waist. Keep your knees straight but not locked. Start with your hands on your hips.

- Stop when your torso is parallel with the floor. Slowly arch your back…and relax. Draw your right shoulder up toward your head…relax. Draw your left shoulder up toward your head…relax.

- Continue lowering your torso toward the floor. Let your arms drop down. *Do not force this motion.* Just slowly allow the muscles all the way up the backs of your legs to stretch.

- Return to standing.

Repeat each stretch until that part of your body feels limber and stiffness and soreness have left.

When stretching, it's important to remember to keep breathing. To this simple, beginning regimen, you will add other stretches to benefit the muscles inside and on the front of your legs.

Strategy #3: Rub It Out (Massage)

Massage can have a very important place in headache and migraine relief. Why? Because it's a strategy that actually touches (no pun intended) the body, mind, and spirit.

Many parents recognize the power of massage instinctively. If you have ever gently rubbed the arm or back of a fussy, upset, or agitated child…and watched them settle down and even fall asleep, you understand the power of massage. This type of "light" massage draws the body, mind, and spirit into a "distracted from all cares" kind of single focus…inducing deep relaxation.

There are different types of massage, from the "light touch" massage just described, to the more vigorous, "deep muscle" massages. You will want to carefully experiment—until you find the level of massage that is vigorous enough to release your muscle tensions without causing undue discomfort—to discover which kind works for you.

Obviously, this is a strategy for which you need a partner. If you do not have one ready-at-hand, you can check your local telephone listings to locate a Licensed Massage Therapist (LMT) in your area. Or call: The American Massage Therapy Association: (847) 864-0123.

If you have a private partner, you can benefit greatly by using one of the excellent massage books now on the market. Recommended reading: *Massage for Dummies: A Reference for the Rest of Us®* by Steve Capellini and Michel Van Welden (Indianapolis: Hungry Minds, Inc.).

To increase the benefits of your massage experience, add:

- **Your favorite relaxing music.** Ask your LMT if he or she has a sound system and if you can bring your favorite tapes or CDs along. This can help calm the mind.

- **Aromatherapy.** Check out the list of headache-releasing essential oils in Chapter 6. Using them will help to encourage deep breathing, which further enhances the physical effects of the massage.

- **Spiritual Scriptures.** Some people benefit spiritually by listening to scriptures on tape during massage. They find that
  verses they have read many times before—such as the
  Psalms—take on new and deeper meaning when they listen
  to them during this experience.

Today, many doctors and counselors are recommending that
clients with long-standing problems—from emotional pain and
confusion, to mental ruts—try massage therapy in an effort to
release stresses lodged in the body. Sometimes they may recom-
mend a special form of massage therapy known as "body work."

Body work is done by specially trained therapists, using the
theory that we sometimes associate pain with a certain part of the
body. When we experience later distress, the theory goes, that part
of the body will tense up, and in time, it may "lock up," leaving us
with chronic muscle tensions, injuries, and postural problems.
These locked muscles can trigger, among other physical problems,
headaches and migraines.

You may wish to consider using "body work" if you suspect you
are carrying painful or injurious emotions from past experiences,
such as anger, fear, or unresolved grief.

Strategy #4: Unlock Muscle Knots (Acupressure)

And then there are simple muscle knots....

A high percentage of headaches, and many migraines as well,
are triggered by tension stored in the muscles. Stress is still the cul-
prit behind this condition, whether it's stress from physical overwork, the stress generated by mental tensions, or the kind generated
from even deeper inside by some buried spiritual stress.

When this happens a muscle will seize up, or spasm, pinching
the nerves that pass through it. In fact, one muscle in spasm may
trigger a spasm in an adjacent muscle, setting off a chain reaction.
So, for instance, a muscle in your midback may spasm, triggering
spasms in your whole upper back, or along one side of your back.
The result is that this part of your back turns into a series of hard
and painful muscle knots...which radiates pain up into your neck,

around your temples…and squeezes your forehead and crown in an excruciating grip.

Often this stress can be released just by locating "trigger points" in the muscles and exerting carefully aimed, constant pressure, until the spasm relaxes.

"Acupressure" is the name for this practice. And it's one of those wonderful, natural pain-release strategies you can do for yourself, just about anytime or anywhere. It can be used to prevent a muscle-tension headache or migraine when you feel it coming on. Or to release one when it strikes quickly—for instance, when a cold draft or lifting something heavy causes a muscle to seize up.

Do This:

Use these charts to help you locate possible muscle spasms the next time you experience a headache or migraine. (You may be surprised to find that your pain can radiate from a tiny muscle knot hidden under a cheekbone…or way down in your lower back, even as low as the upper part of the buttocks.)

1. Begin by checking your facial muscles. People suffering from sinus headaches, especially, will find relief by using this part of the strategy. Use your thumbs and index fingers to explore your facial muscles. While exerting a bit of pressure, explore the bony ridge above your eye socket. Then move to the bridge of your nose…and from there move out and along your brow. (**See figure 1 / 1.**)

Next, explore the underside of your cheekbones on both sides …then down along the front side of your jawbone. (**See figure 1 / 2.**)

Figure 1

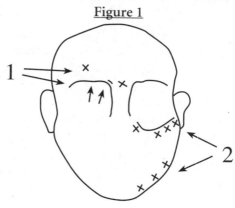

2. Continue…checking your whole head, and then your neck.
Starting beside each eye, work back along the depressions that form
your temples…back to the top of your ears. Use a small circling
motion and press as you move your fingers. (**See figure 2 / 1.**)
(**Figure 2 / 2** is a side view of the cheekbones and jawline, to better
help you locate the trigger points there.)

Next, exert pressure on the back of your skull, about an inch
behind your earlobes. Move down to the base of your skull…and
also gently press along both sides of the cervical vertebrae in your
neck. (**See figure 2 / 3.**)

Then, starting below the corners of your jaw, move your fingers
down the long muscles on either side of your neck. (**See figure 2 / 4.**)

<u>Figure 2</u>

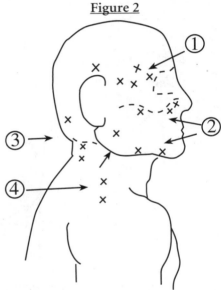

3. Now reach around to feel the muscles behind your shoul-
ders…in the whole upper back area. Raking, shoveling, typing,
lifting…a whole range of activities can cause the muscles of the
upper back and shoulders to seize up. If you are not limber enough
to do this, try leaning against a doorjamb or the corner of a wall, to
locate possible muscle knots in this area.

(**Figure 3 / 1** gives you another view of the trigger points at the
back of your head and along your neck.)

Feel along the upper part of your shoulder for the trigger points there. (**See figure 3 / 2.**)

You will find a whole series of headache/migraine trigger points located all around the edges, and on top of, your shoulder blades. (**See figure 3 / 3.**)

For the final part of this step, feel along both sides of your spine. Begin just above your midback and move down to the backside of your diaphragm. (**See figure 3 / 4.**)

<u>Figure 3</u>

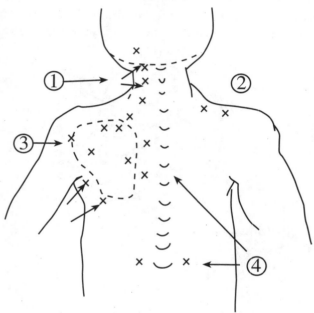

4. *This step can give you some real surprises. Very dull headaches and overall achiness can also be triggered from way down in the lower back and the buttocks.*

Apply pressure to the lower back just above the beltline...and move down about two inches to the "spines" at the back of your pelvis. (**See figure 4 / 1.**)

Finally, use your thumbs to press into the ridge along the top and back of your pelvis...and move out to your hip sockets. (**See figure 4 / 2.**)

Figure 4

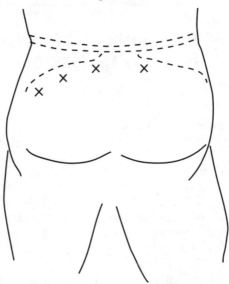

Because these muscles are larger, the knots in this particular area can be worked out better in this manner:

Sit on the floor and cross one ankle over the opposite knee. Grab the bent knee in your hands…and slowly, gently pull up…feeling the muscles in your hips and buttocks stretch…and the pain-causing knots release.

Deep-muscle massage therapies, such as Rolfing or Hellerwork, are a combination of massage and acupressure. Some headache sufferers may find them helpful, while others may find that these experiences are too painful…and even trigger their headaches.

If you want to find a Rolfing or Hellerwork practitioner near you, contact:

Rolf Institute: 1-800-530-8875

or

Hellerwork: 1-800-392-3900

THE ALEXANDER TECHNIQUE OR FELDENKRAIS METHOD

∾

This pain-release strategy is based on the idea that increased awareness of what's going on in our bodies can help us locate and release physical trigger points of pain. This makes it a great option for headache and migraine sufferers.

Like many bodywork techniques, the Alexander method is hard to describe. Essentially, you are taught how to focus in on the parts of your body until you detect tension. Then, by using different postures or movements, you learn how to release the tension or "restriction" and feel the relaxation or "freedom" return.

To find a practitioner of this great and healing technique near you, call:

North American Society of Teachers of the Alexander Technique: 1-800-473-0620 or Feldenkrais Guild: 1-800-775-2118.

Strategy #6: Non-Impact Aerobics (NIA)

As we've discussed, sudden pressure changes within the circulatory system can be a serious problem for headache and migraine sufferers. So can jarring, high-impact motions.

Non-Impact Aerobics (NIA) is a great strategy for increasing circulation and exercising tension out of your muscles *without* the stress of regular aerobics or calisthenics.

NIA increases metabolism, respiration, and heart rate. Studies have shown that it also helps your body to release hormones that trigger the deep relaxation response...instead of the stress hormones produced by high-impact workouts which remain in your system and cause muscle knotting later as your body cools down and circulation slows.

Many NIA instructors also encourage good mental conditioning by the use of simple, guided imagery. This can help you reach a positive frame of mind, which, of course, is another key to releasing the deep relaxation hormones. (If you prefer, you can provide your own meditational experience using music you enjoy or a tape of scriptures from your spiritual tradition.)

Do This:

- Check with local community centers, gyms, or health clubs to sign up for NIA classes.

- Purchase a taped version of the sacred writings of your religious tradition, or a tape of positive affirmation. These are available in many large bookstores and through on-line tape and booksellers.

- As you engage in NIA routines, meditate on the truths that speak to you and allow your mind to be renewed, your spirit made lighter...and your physical stresses to drain away.

Strategy #7: "Walk Away" from a Headache

Walking is still one of the best nonstressing strategies we can use to release physical tensions. Walking gently raises the heart-rate and oxygenates the blood by restoring proper breathing. Done in the right frame of mind, it can restore a relaxed mental and spiritual state, too.

For a truly great walking experience...

Do This:

1. Choose two or three walking routes. Choose one short distance (10-minute walk), one mid-range (20-minute), and one longer course (30 minutes or more). This will give you changes in scenery and options to choose from depending on how much time you have.

2. Buy good walking shoes. Shoes that can "breathe" and support your instep and ankles are the best choice. Expensive isn't necessarily better, but don't cheap-out and make your feet and legs suffer either.

YOGA

∽

Many western people are discovering the vast health benefits of yoga that eastern cultures have enjoyed for thousands of years. Yoga increases strength and flexibility and only gradually increases your heart rate. Because its motions are smooth, not jarring, it doesn't place sudden strains on the cardiovascular system, *and* it encourages proper breathing, yoga is an excellent choice of exercise for many headache and migraine sufferers.

There are various types of yoga. But the basic kind—which involves stretching, holding certain postures, focus on breathing—can be easily learned with the aid of videos you can use at home. You are also likely to find instructional courses offered at local gyms and community centers.

For those who are concerned about the "eastern" flavor of yoga—that is, those who are not interested in learning or practicing eastern philosophy—have no fear. Many instructors teach yoga strictly for its physical health benefits, without the metaphysical content.

3. Get your walking rhythm and your pulse up. Focus on your stride and your breathing, until you've reached a pace that encourages proper breathing...but not panting. (See Strategy #1.)

4. Focus your mind. You can begin by focusing on your breathing. Or you may want to focus on "positive" thoughts. Or you may want to spend the time praying. The main point is to unburden your inner being as you allow your body to walk off physical stress.

5. Very important: Slow your pace for the last part of your walk. It's not a good idea to burn it up past the finish line...and then chug inside and drop into a chair. As your walk comes to an end, allow your body a *10- or 15-minute slowdown period.* This lets your respiration and circulation return gradually to normal resting rates.

Remember, you do not want to stress your circulatory system by suddenly starting or stopping any exercise or activity.

Listening to Your Body

"Biofeedback" is a fancy word for paying attention to what's going on in your physical body. If you have ever had the sudden realization that you've been clenching your teeth or making a fist without even realizing it, you have some idea what this is about. Much of the time, our attention is so riveted on life all *around* us that we lose touch with what's going on *in* us.

As you may have noted, the physical strategies for headache and migraine relief have an awareness-raising component to them. That's because it's very important that you work out physical tensions *and* at the same time learn how to "listen to your body."

If you try these strategies *mindfully* paying attention to your body's actions and reactions, you will vastly increase your chances of releasing headaches and migraines that are the result of body stress—and also increase your chances of preventing them.

You can gain only by learning how to be more in tune with your body.

8

Balance

Y ou set out in the morning to knock out the items on your day's schedule. You're doing great, getting a lot done...and the headache begins. Before you know it, all you want is a quiet room with a sofa or bed, and an ice pack to help soothe the aching beat in your temples.

In time, you realize: This is the way life is going to be. You're not thrilled about it, but you start to take your headaches and migraines in stride.

You learn when it's time to quit...before a dull throb turns into a killer headache.

You also learn when and how to just keep trudging through. You learn that you can "play hurt." You can still get a lot done even when it feels like some malignant entity is hammering on your skull.

In time, you pride yourself on the way you've learned to accommodate the headaches and migraines. You think you've taken the bad card you were dealt and figured out how to play it well.

But is that true?

What you may not notice is that pain seems to be taking over the center of your world. It's becoming a sort of dark polestar around which your personal world moves. In the back of your mind you're always planning for it, mentally angling around places, times, people, or situations that might trigger it.

Centering on Wellness

To add a final perspective...It's important for each of us to step back and take an honest look at our whole life. When we do, we may begin to see headaches and migraines, and our efforts to avoid them, have actually taken over and become the very thing we've centered our lives around.

There is a difference, of course, between taking pain into account...and letting it take over the very core of our lives. When we're plagued with an affliction that causes so much distress, it's easy for us to make pain the central issue and not even be aware we're doing so.

Take a moment right now and ask yourself out of concern that you might trigger a headache or migraine...

- **Do you frequently excuse yourself from getting healthy exercise? hard work? celebrations? social obligations?**

- **Do you think of yourself as "impaired"—"less able" or even "less than" other people?**

- **Do you hear, or read about, strategies for releasing yourself from headaches or migraines and think, *These will never work for me*?**

There is no doubt the pain of headaches and migraines is excruciating. When it strikes, there is not much you can do but retreat from stress and seek relief. But...

The real question we're asking here is:

- **Have you rearranged your whole life around the avoidance of pain—made pain and sickness the center of your life?**

Only you can answer that question. And there is no shame or guilt if your answer is, "Yes, I guess I have."

The only reason for raising the issue here is to help you make a new choice. That is, the choice to stop centering your life around your problem and instead center it around the experience of wellness.

Wellness...from Balance

When we speak of centering our lives around wellness, we're not talking about becoming "health nuts" or just refocusing on "doing whatever it takes to feel better." We're talking about something much broader and deeper than that. We're talking about learning to live in balance, paying attention to all aspects of our being.

For some, this very idea will seem awkward and new and uncomfortable. You may think, "If I pay *that* much attention to myself, won't I just become incredibly self-centered?" The answer is: If you're already self-centered, the kind of balance we're suggesting will make you *less* self-focused and more self-giving.

What does it mean, then, to pay attention to our whole being and live in balance? There is no "formula" for achieving balance, frankly. But here are several practical ways you can make the move toward wellness and balance.

Make a space in your daily life for the things that will keep you well in body, mind, and spirit.

For most of us, this begins with paying attention to our personal schedule. Too often we let everyone else's demands and agendas crowd out what we really need to do to stay well ourselves.

Making a space in our lives for all aspects of our being means setting aside time to:

- *commune with, and be inspired by, the awesomeness of God (a.k.a. worship)*

- *stretch our spirits by taking stock of how we are living in relation to our deepest values, especially in relation to other people and to our work*

- *grow our mind, by expanding our thinking with new and challenging ideas*

- *strengthen and limber up our bodies with exercise and play*

- *eat well and rest well*

Set aside time, at least monthly, to go deeper...and really examine the workings of your life.

Most of us can't give a lot of time to healthy self-examination. And yet, that's what overall wellness and balance requires. When you do set aside time for a more careful look at your life, these questions can help you get a firmer hold on wellness and a balanced life:

- What if I paid more careful attention to my relationship with God?

- What if I sought God's mind, heart, and will for my life more carefully? And what if I followed it—where would it lead me? What if I lived more carefully in tune with my values and my conscience? What if I gave more time and energy to my best life goals and less energy to satisfying my personal demands for immediate gratification?

- What if I saw all of my life, and my own self, as a gift from God?

- What if I saw my mind as a gift from God and decided to develop a healthier mental life?

- What if I learned to discipline my mind: to turn it away from all forms of negative or degrading thinking? What if I opened my mind to the possibilities in life instead of dwelling on the "impossibilities"?

- What if I saw my heart, my emotions, and my relationships as a gift from God?

- What if I decided to listen and understand more in my relationships? What if I decided to learn what it means to connect with other people through empathy and caring? What would my relationships be like if I criticized and gossiped less? If I was less caustic, critical, competitive? What if I learned how to see the good and genuinely encouraged and built up other people more?

- What if I learned to say "No" when I need to say no…and stuck to my decision…and stopped resenting what I do for others? And what if I said "Yes" wholeheartedly when I want to say yes…and started throwing enthusiasm and energy into it when I help other people?

- Suppose I begin to treat my body as a gift from God— because it's the only physical home my mind and spirit are ever going to have?

Would I eat differently? Less? Better? Are there substances I run through my stomach, blood, and lungs…that I'd stop using? Would I make just a little more effort to keep it in shape, so I can enjoy living here as long as possible? Would I rest more?

Finally,

> ### *Set aside time once a year to review your life's course…what ground you've covered in the past twelve months…and where you want to go in the twelve that lie just ahead.*

Life is full of transitions:

The season for staying at our current job ends.

A longstanding relationship goes through change and upheaval.

Our body's needs are different now than they were a year ago.

Our attitudes and beliefs, deep beneath the surface of daily living, shift and change.

All this is part of being human.

The problem is, we are creatures of habit. When life changes …and even when mental, emotional, and spiritual changes occur in us…we often remain in the rut of doing exactly what we've always done. Oddly enough, we can miss the transitions we're going through and wind up living way out of touch with ourselves.

This losing touch with ourselves creates big and deep tensions...the way tectonic plates in the earth grind against each other before an earthquake. Some of us wait until a health crisis or a tragedy wakes us up. And then we reevaluate and change.

A better way to live is to take a more active part in our life as we grow and change. It is to recognize shifts in attitude, changes in belief, new thoughts...also to make a place in our life for new needs.

Harder, perhaps, is the need to let go of things that no longer have usefulness or meaning. Then courage becomes the power that moves us on in our journey toward a new sense of wellness and balance.

Some people make annual pilgrimages to retreat centers or monasteries...some to secluded cabins in the woods or cottages on the seashore. Others simply clear their schedule for a long weekend. What they discover is that taking time to get the long view of what's behind, and what might lie before, gives them perspective and motivation. More than that, it gives them that all-important spark of drive and hope that by being more mindful of what's important, *the time that lies ahead* might become their best time yet.

My Hope for You

It's my hope that you have found within this book practical strategies to help relieve your headache and migraine pain.

And along with that, it's my prayer that you will in fact take time to seek wellness and a balanced life in the fullest sense. And that you'll enjoy life as the great gift it is.

The New Nature Institute

The New Nature Institute was founded in 1999 for the purpose of exploring the connection between personal health and wellness and spirituality, with the Hebrew-Christian tradition as its spiritual foundation.

Drawing upon this tradition, the Institute supports the belief that humankind is created in the image of God. We are each body, mind, and spirit and so intricately connected that each aspect of our being affects the other. If one aspect suffers, our whole being suffers; if all aspects are being supported, we will enjoy a greater sense of well-being.

For this reason, the Institute engages in ongoing research in order to provide up-to-date information that supports a "whole-person" approach to wellness. Most especially, research is focused on the natural approaches to wellness that support health and vitality in the body, mind, and spirit.

Healthy Body, Healthy Soul is a series of books intended to complement treatment plans provided by healthcare professionals. They are not meant to be used in place of professional consultations and/or treatment plans.

Along with creating written materials, the New Nature Institute also presents seminars, workshops, and retreats on a range of topics relating to spirituality and wellness. These can be tailored for corporate, spiritual community, or general community settings.

For information contact:
    The New Nature Institute
    Attn: David Hazard
    P.O. Box 568
    Round Hill, Virginia 20142
    (540) 338-7032
    Exangelos@aol.com